BRAVING A VIRAL STORM

'A riveting narration of how India overcame a global catastrophe. The authors have taken a very positive approach of highlighting India's collective resolve in battling the Covid-19 pandemic. An authoritative journey of the Indian innovative vaccination story. A must read for everyone who believes in India and it's scientific minds.'

—Dr Krishna Ella

Executive Chairman, Bharat Biotech International Limited

'A brilliant, must-read account of one of independent India's greatest achievements—to have vaccinated a billion Indians within a year, twice over.'

—Anand Ranganathan

Professor, Special Centre for Molecular Medicine,
Jawaharlal Nehru University,
Author and Columnist

'*Braving a Viral Storm* is the perfect encapsulation of how a confident India proved the world wrong. The book celebrates the power of our self-belief and nudges us to be proud of our achievements.'

—Vivek Ranjan Agnihotri

Award-winning Film Producer and Director

BRAVING A VIRAL STORM

India's Covid-19 Vaccine Story

AASHISH CHANDORKAR
and **SURAJ SUDHIR**

RUPA

First published by
Rupa Publications India Pvt. Ltd 2023
7/16, Ansari Road, Daryaganj
New Delhi 110002

Sales Centres:

Allahabad Bengaluru Chennai
Hyderabad Jaipur Kathmandu
Kolkata Mumbai

P-ISBN: 978-93-5520-974-0
E-ISBN: 978-93-5520-975-7

First impression 2023

10 9 8 7 6 5 4 3 2 1

Printed in India

Aashish Chandorkar dedicates this book to India, that is Bharat, a civilizational nation that has weathered many storms and will successfully navigate many more.

Suraj Sudhir dedicates this book to the spirit of India, its strength and resilience in the face of all odds.

CONTENTS

FOREWORD

I write this foreword to the book covering the monumental success story of India's Covid-19 vaccination on the day India has achieved the target of administering 2 billion vaccine doses. This milestone has been accomplished in 18 months after India launched its vaccination programme.

Two billion vaccine doses—doesn't it sound surreal? When we were in the middle of the Covid-19 pandemic in 2020, India's capacity to run a nationwide vaccination programme targeted at adults was questioned, lampooned and prejudged to be a failure. There were suggestions that India may take 10 years to vaccinate its entire population.

It was not just the Indian government but also the Indians who were subjected to veiled ridicule, assuming that they will not understand the importance of vaccination. And yet, here we are in a country where more than 90 per cent of the adults are fully vaccinated and more than 95 per cent of the adults have taken at least one dose of the Covid-19 vaccine at the time of writing.

How did India prove its critics wrong? The answer is very simple and, in fact, can be explained in one word—trust. India trusted the leadership of Prime Minister Shri Narendra Modi, who in his eight-year-long tenure has taken the country from strength to strength, while earning the love, affection, respect and, most importantly, unflinching trust of 1.4 billion Indians.

The leadership demonstrated by the PM in steering India through the course of the Covid-19 pandemic has been exemplary. His vision for India to invest time, effort and financial resources early on in potential vaccine candidates paid off. It was this vision and conviction he put in India's scientific and research talent which ensured that India became *aatmanirbhar* (self-reliant) when it came to ensuring vaccine availability, access and affordability in the country.

This Triple A rating—availability, access and affordability—is a matter of pride and immense satisfaction for India. We have seen countries around the world struggle and fight for their requirement of Covid-19 vaccines. Several global leaders have had to plead with private pharmaceutical companies to give them vaccines, often in lieu of accepting ignominious terms and conditions.

India, on the other hand, has not just fought the virus successfully, it has done so with its head held high. This is a story of India's courage, conviction and collective efforts, and it stands out in the world, despite the inherent complexity of our country.

India has also initiated several measures to ensure that our scientific heft and capability are deployed to counter any future health crises in a coordinated and effective manner. The government has worked on institutionalizing the learning from this pandemic in terms of research and development, skills and training initiatives, investments in cutting-edge medical facilities and creating the right social safety nets for the most vulnerable sections of society.

This story needed to be told, and I am glad that the authors of this book, Aashish Chandorkar and Suraj Sudhir, have taken up this task of national importance. Our vibrant democracy sometimes tends to be hypercritical about our smallest failures and does not fully recognize and celebrate even the biggest of our achievements. This book plugs this important gap—it displays the best of India and implores the readers to honour India's many successes.

The authors have written a factually enlightening account of India's strong pushback against the Covid-19 pandemic, seeking to inform the readers of the true challenges faced by the country. The authors have spent precious time in speaking to various experts in this field in India and around the world to provide balanced and comprehensive perspectives to India's vaccination story.

It is a matter of great joy and relief that India's vaccination success, led by the untiring efforts of Prime Minister Shri Narendra Modi, is being told in real time, while the memories of the pandemic as well as our fight back against it are fresh in the public memory.

Dr Mansukh Mandaviya
Minister of Health and Family Welfare,
and Chemical and Fertilizers, Government of India
New Delhi
17 July 2022

HOPE DAWNS

'*Laga bhi di...aur pata bhi nahi chala* (You already administered [the vaccine], I didn't even realize),' PM Narendra Modi remarked light-heartedly to Sister P. Niveda, when she inoculated him.[1]

Sister Niveda, originally from Puducherry, and Sister Rosamma Anil,[2] hailing from Kerala, were called upon on the morning of 1 March 2021 to administer the first dose of the Covid-19 vaccine to the PM.

It was the day India's fight against Covid-19 moved from containment measures, like lockdowns, to ring-fencing the population from the virus. Although the vaccination drive against Covid-19 had kicked off earlier in the year, on 16 January, on 1 March, the vaccination drive for all Indians over 60 and over 45 with comorbidities was started.

PM Modi took the 6-km journey from 7, Lok Kalyan Marg, his official residence, to the All India Institute of Medical Sciences (AIIMS) early in the morning. Sister Niveda administered Covaxin to the PM. Covaxin, Bharat Biotech's home-grown inactivated-virus-based vaccine, had been developed in partnership with the Indian Council of Medical Research (ICMR).

PM Modi taking a truly 'Made in India' vaccine and publicizing the event, urging individuals to participate in the vaccination drive, was not coincidental. His choice of vaccine as well as his clear message[3] was to prove instrumental in kicking off a long battle, which India eventually won.

But this was not a fait accompli on the said date. India was to soon find out that it was fighting against not just a virus, which was only 50–150 nanometre in size, the country was also going to face an information warfare at an industrial scale.

1

DARK CLOUDS ENGULF THE WORLD

The human mind is wired in such a way that it worries about events that are likely to occur in the near future and likely to cause exclusive proximate harm, or both. A potential pandemic would fall in neither category. There were no forthcoming pandemics, except in academic analyses or in Hollywood movies. Even when there were signs of global diseases, like Severe Acute Respiratory Syndrome (SARS) in 2002, H1N1 influenza, popularly called swine flu, in 2009, or Middle East Respiratory Syndrome (MERS) in 2012, the impact was either geographically limited or the morbidity rates were nothing to cause long-term anxiety.

Vaclav Smil, a Canadian economic analyst, wrote in his book, *Global Catastrophes and Trends*, in 2008:

> The likelihood of another influenza pandemic during the next 50 years is virtually 100%, but quantifying probabilities of mild, moderate, or severe events remains largely a matter of speculation because we simply do not know how pathogenic a new virus will be and what age categories it will preferentially attack. Assessing the most likely extent of morbidity and mortality is even more challenging.[1]

Smil's concerns remained largely academic. One of his avid followers, William Henry Gates III, popularly known as Bill Gates, who moved towards philanthropy, had been warning about pandemics. In his 2015 TED Talk, Gates said:

> As awful as this epidemic has been, the next one could be much worse. The world is simply not prepared to deal with a disease—an especially virulent flu, for example—that infects large numbers of people very quickly. Of all the things that could kill 10 million people or more, by far the most likely is an epidemic.[2]

Gates was speaking about the Ebola epidemic that had broken out in West Africa. But Ebola's impact was always limited. It did not spread fast and wide enough to cause a global mayhem. Hence, Gates' views on pandemics, which he continued to express throughout the last decade, remained a subject of curiosity at most.

Meanwhile, Hollywood had chipped in with creative, forward-thinking movies in recent years. The 2011 movie, *Contagion*, directed by Steven Soderbergh, and the 2016 movie, *Pandemic*, directed by John Suits, involved heroic doctors saving a beleaguered world.

The voices talking about a 1918 Spanish-Flu-style pandemic had been growing increasingly loud. Jeremy Konyndyk, former director of U.S. Agency for International Development's (USAID) Office of U.S. Foreign Disaster Assistance (OFDA), talked about how the United States (US) was not prepared to handle a pandemic in 2017.[3] Robert G. Webster, a researcher at the University of Otago, published a book, *Flu Hunter: Unlocking the Secrets of a Virus*, just before the world heard of the Covid-19 pandemic.[4]

Dr Krishna Ella, chairman and managing director of Bharat Biotech, was in New Delhi on 3 December 2019, launching Rotavac 5D, a new variant of their oral rotavirus vaccine, which could be administered in a smaller dosage and stored at higher temperatures compared to the previous products. It was also Dr Ella's marriage anniversary,[5] but the product launch meant he could not celebrate the day with his wife. From Delhi, he had to fly to Bengaluru for the Global Technology Summit, organized by Carnegie India.

With the helplessness born of the professional demands encroaching on his personal life, Dr Ella spent that evening working for his panel discussion on pandemic preparedness. He was sharing the stage with Frederik Kristénsen, deputy chief executive officer (CEO) at the Coalition for Epidemic Preparedness Innovations (CEPI), and Gagandeep Kang, the chairperson and executive director of the Translational Health Science and Technology Institute (THSTI) in Bengaluru.

His remarks[6] at Carniege India Global Technology Summit 2019, held at The Leela Palace on 5 December had an air of premonition. He warned that epidemics and pandemics were always round the corner and likely to start off from developing countries and then spread further. He emphasized that the conferences like the one he was speaking at would stop getting organized if a pandemic was to hit the world. He stressed that it was important to develop vaccines, as they protected not just human life but also economies and societies from the probable wrath of a pandemic. Dr Ella jokingly also added that even Bengaluru's information technology (IT) industry could not predict epidemics using big data and should, in fact, be thankful to vaccine makers for warding off the threat of pathogens.

He was to be proven right in a month.

The World Comes to Know

When the Covid-19 virus actually started spreading, it took the world by storm. The theories had not prepared anyone for the deadly onslaught.

How and when the SARS 2019 novel coronavirus, earlier dubbed SARS-CoV-2 or 2019-nCoV, appeared is still a matter of research. With the benefit of hindsight and through what is perhaps one of the most persistent human research efforts in history, we now know that the virus had been identified in Wuhan, China, by November 2019.

As per a report by the *South China Morning Post*, the virus was known to the Chinese authorities by 17 November 2019. The Chinese government records showed that the first person to contract the virus may have been a 55-year-old resident of the Hubei province, but the authorities could not identify 'patient zero'. The article claimed that the Chinese authorities had identified 266 individuals as impacted by the virus in November 2019.[7]

A Chinese doctor named Dr Li Wenliang died of the infection caused by the novel coronavirus in early February 2020. He had tried to warn his fellow doctors about the virus back in December 2019. The British Broadcasting Corporation (BBC) published a story about his bravery in February 2020, highlighting the severity of the virus.[8]

Much later, in November 2021, Michael Worobey, a scientist at the University of Arizona, conducted painstaking research to also arrive at the conclusion that the earliest cases of the novel coronavirus could be traced back to November 2019.[9] His research showed that cases of pneumonia were known to have been present in individuals connected with the Huanan Seafood Wholesale Market in Wuhan. The doctors in Wuhan had known of such cases since December 2019.

On their part, the Chinese public health authorities asked hospitals in the said region to report any new cases of pneumonia on 30 December 2019. On 1 January 2020, the authorities shut down the Huanan market fearing another SARS-like public health outbreak.[10] Later, on 11 January 2020, the Chinese authorities dated the earliest known case of the mysterious pneumonia to 8 December 2019.[11]

The exact nature of the origin of the virus will continue to be a matter of investigation. Whether the virus was transmitted from animals, like bats, to human beings or whether it leaked from a bioresearch lab in Wuhan will be a matter of both scientific studies as well as wild conjectures for years to come. But what is perhaps clear is that the global response did lag by a few weeks, despite the information being available by early January 2020.

The World Health Organization (WHO) had taken note of the rising pneumonia cases in Wuhan and put in place an Incident Management Support Team by 1 January 2020. The United Nations (UN) agency responsible for international public health shared an update on 4 January 2020 on its Twitter feed, reporting a cluster of mysterious pneumonia cases in Wuhan.[12]

That the public health emergency was already getting serious was reflected in the fact that the WHO had, by 10 January 2020, already advised all countries on how to detect, test and manage potential cases.[13]

Things were moving at a frenetic pace. The Chinese researchers shared a draft sequence of the novel coronavirus on 11 January 2020. This was reported by the journal *Science*, stating, 'Scientists worried about China's lack of transparency about a month-old outbreak of pneumonia in the city of Wuhan breathed a sigh of relief today, after a consortium of researchers published a draft genome of the newly discovered coronavirus suspected of causing the outbreak.'[14]

However, the virus was already keeping well ahead of science. On 13 January 2020, the first case of Covid-19 was detected in Thailand.[15] National boundaries were far too easy for the virus to cross.

A study published in the medical journal *The Lancet* on 24 January 2020 warned about human-to-human transmission of this virus. The summary interpretation of this study said, 'Our findings are consistent with person-to-person transmission of this novel coronavirus in hospital and family settings, and the reports of infected travellers in other geographical regions.'[16]

However, while the research work prior to the publishing of the study in *The Lancet* was happening, the WHO shared on its Twitter feed that there was no evidence of human-to-human transmission of the novel coronavirus. This statement was first made on 12 January 2020[17] and later repeated on 14 January 2020[18].

The International Committee on Taxonomy of Viruses (ICTV) named the virus as SARS-CoV-2 on 11 February 2020. On the same day, the WHO decided to call the virus 'Covid-19' for ease of reference.[19]

By now, the virulent pathogen was already making its way through the world. After Thailand and Japan, South Korea and the US were next. By the end of January, the virus had reached Asia, Europe and North America. In February, countries in Africa and South America also saw cases of Covid-19.[20]

Covid-19 Comes to India

India reported its first case of Covid-19 on 30 January 2020. The first-known Indian patient was a student at Wuhan University who had returned to Thrissur in Kerala after the outbreak in Wuhan.[21] The virus claimed its first victim in India on 12 March 2020 in Karnataka. A 76-year-old man, who had returned from Saudi Arabia, died in Kalbauragi.[22]

However, after the first case was discovered, the next month was relatively quiet. While countries like the US and Italy had been gripped by the virus, along with China, India was preparing for the oncoming onslaught. Dr V.K. Paul, working with the NITI Aayog, and Prof. K. VijayRaghavan, then principal scientific advisor to the PM, had started working on understanding the virus and its spread, which was the immediate concern for a large and relatively resource-constrained society and economy like India.[23]

By March, the virus started entrenching itself in India. The spread in India was rapid—a foregone conclusion, given the size of the population and deep interstate as well as international linkages. By 23 March 2020, lockdowns were imposed in 20 states and union territories (UTs).[24] As different states and UTs took their own initial measures to combat the unknown, the Union government stepped in to bring a uniform initial response to the pandemic.

The country had to be prepared for a lockdown. Given the complex interlinkages within the Indian socio-economic system, this was not going to be easy. Just explaining the idea to people would require a high degree of persuasion. PM Modi appeared on television for a national address at 7.00 p.m. on 19 March. He asked Indians to observe a 'janata curfew' on 22 March from 7.00 a.m. to 9.00 p.m. The intent was to create a sense of ownership in society towards the rapid spread of the virus and follow the stringent lockdown that was to come.[25]

PM Modi announced a national lockdown on 24 March via yet another televised address.[26] He was direct and emphatic in the address. He recognized that many states had already taken their initial measures, but added that, based on expert advice, a national intervention was necessary.

> In the last two days, several parts of the country have been put under lockdown. These efforts by State Governments should be taken very seriously.
>
> Keeping in mind health sector experts and experiences of other countries, the nation is about to take a very important decision today. From 12 midnight today the entire country, please listen carefully, the entire country shall go under complete lockdown. In order to protect the country, and each of its citizens, from midnight tonight, a complete ban is being imposed on people from stepping out of their homes.
>
> Every State of the country, every Union Territory, every district, every municipality, every village, every street, every locality is being put under lockdown. This is in effect a type of curfew only. A few levels more than Janata-Curfew, it is more stringent.[27]

This 21-day lockdown was to prove instrumental in giving India the required time to mount the initial response to the pandemic. When the virus had hit India, there were very little provisions even for basic protective equipment.[28] The national lockdown was intended to slow down the spread of the virus across the country, which could have otherwise burdened the healthcare systems across the country.

The World Scrambles to Act

The director general of WHO, Dr Tedros Adhanom Ghebreyesus announced on 11 March 2020 in Geneva that the number of cases, deaths and affected countries was expected to increase in the weeks to come. Dr Ghebreyesus said, 'We have never before seen a pandemic sparked by a coronavirus. This is the first pandemic caused by a coronavirus.'[29] He could not have been more prescient. By mid-March 2022, the virus had claimed more than 6 million lives globally,[30] with India losing more than half a million individuals to it.[31]

As the virus ravaged unprepared countries and economies, scientists globally had already started thinking about how to combat it. Based in Oslo, Norway, CEPI was the first international organization to announce plans of developing vaccines to tackle Covid-19. On 23 January 2020, it announced that it would start three different vaccine development programmes, involving its existing partnerships with Inovio, The University of Queensland in Brisbane, Australia and a new partnership with the American pharmaceuticals and biotechnology firm, Moderna, and the National Institute of Allergy and Infectious Diseases (NIAID) in the US.[32]

Around the same time, China's National Health Commission recommended using Human Immunodeficiency Virus or HIV drugs as a potential treatment against Covid-19. The Chinese Center for Disease Control and Prevention also started working on a potential vaccine candidate against Covid-19.[33]

At that time, the Covid-19 virus was ahead of the capabilities of global science. But the global race to tame, if not defeat, the virus was truly on.

2

THE ONE-MILLILITRE ELIXIR

Human history is one of fortitude. Diseases ravaged vast swathes of populations before modern medical science started to mount a predictive and stiff resistance against them. Epidemics have not just been routine, they have also been events of mass destruction at every occurrence.

The historical usage of the term 'pandemic' has been relatively infrequent compared to the term 'epidemic'. While there have been relatively fewer pandemics in history, the human species has encountered several epidemics. The earliest ones tended to be more localized, as the world was separated by distance.

A pandemic is defined as 'an epidemic occurring worldwide, or over a very wide area, crossing international boundaries and usually affecting a large number of people'.[1] Hence, all pandemics are epidemics, but only some epidemics go on to get classified as pandemics.

In the recent decades, international bodies, like the WHO, have worked on fine-tuning these definitional aspects, which help the member countries classify a disease and its expected severity. The world had not really witnessed a true pandemic after the Spanish Flu of 1918. However, history has not been that kind.

The first epidemic of human history—because it was recorded as such—occurred sometime from 165 AD to 180 AD in the Roman Empire.[2] Named the Antonine Plague or the Plague of Galen after the physician who recorded it, the disease is estimated to have claimed 5 million lives.[3]

The ferocity with which these diseases claimed their victims gradually decreased over time, as the human race became more equipped with medical solutions.

The Bubonic Plague of 1347 took 200 million lives. Smallpox in 1520 claimed 56 million victims. The Plague of Justinian, which may have aided the downfall of the Roman Empire, killed 50 million people in 541 AD. The Spanish Flu that spread at the tail end of First World War, with returning soldiers carrying the virus with them to several parts of the world, killed an estimated 40–50 million individuals.[4] India lost around 40 million people to pandemics of cholera, plague and influenza between 1817 and 1920—it was the most affected country during the time of the outbreak of each of these pandemics.[5] India alone lost 12 million people to the Spanish Flu, which was about 5 per cent of the country's total population then.[6]

There was one commonality in all these instances: the human body's inability to deal with deadly pathogens. There were no known ameliorating methods, let alone cures, for these epidemics. The world largely dealt with the viruses being transmitted between species through a combination of individual resistance, luck and prayers. The mitigating factor was that the spread of the diseases was less global and slower compared to what was witnessed during the Covid-19 pandemic, and the diseases eventually died out on their own.

Although the concept of vaccines had been known in one form or the other since 1000 AD to ancient Chinese, Egyptians and Indians, these were limited and small-scale solutions. It wasn't until Edward Jenner, a British physician born in 1749, conceptualized the idea of a vaccine that the science behind it became commonplace.

Vaccine Development: Ingenuity Triumphs

The term 'vaccine' is derived from *variolae vaccinae*—the term Jenner used to describe the cowpox disease.[7] Jenner's article, published in 1798, 'An Inquiry into the Causes and Effects of the *Variolae Vaccinae*' became the source for the science that went on to save hundreds of millions of lives around the world over the centuries.

The opening words Jenner used in his work almost two and quarter centuries ago may well have been an accurate description of Covid-19 itself. Jenner wrote:

> The deviation of man from the state in which he was originally placed by Nature seems to have proved to him a prolific source of Diseases. From the love of splendour, from the indulgences of luxury, and from his fondness for amusement, he has familiarized himself with a great number of animals, which may not originally have been intended for his associates.[8]

Jenner observed that milkmaids were generally not affected by smallpox. His hypothesis was that the milkmaids had exposure to cowpox, which was a shield against smallpox. He experimented with cowpox-based inoculations on the human subjects of his studies. This 1796 human trial became the bedrock for the science behind vaccinations.[9]

Jenner's work was improved over years of further research. In the year 1807, Bavaria became the first country in the world to introduce compulsory vaccination for smallpox, which was followed by Baden in 1809, Prussia in 1815, Württemberg in 1818 and Sweden in 1816. The German Empire promulgated the Reichs Vaccination Act for the purpose in 1874.[10] The United Kingdom Vaccination Act of 1853 made it mandatory for all children born after 1 August 1853 to be vaccinated for smallpox.[11]

Louis Pasteur, a French chemist and microbiologist, shaped the science of vaccination the way we know it today. In 1885, he developed a vaccine for rabies,[12] which was a serious disease in those times, both by its extent of occurrence as well as impact. Pasteur's work led to doctors beginning to use personal protective equipment (PPE), yet another feature that became a life-saving tool in the early days of the Covid-19 outbreak.

After Pasteur's path-breaking research work, often done at grave personal risk,[13] the science behind vaccination took off. Diseases, such as anthrax, cholera, diphtheria, plague, tetanus, tuberculosis and typhoid, among others, became less severe, as vaccines to protect against their impact were developed.

It was hence natural that the medical world gravitated towards an idea of developing vaccines against Covid-19 as early as January 2020, less than a month into the initial statements made by the Chinese healthcare authorities. However, there was one problem.

Sprinting a Marathon

While the need for vaccination had been well-established, neither the speed nor the scale at which these vaccines were required to contain Covid-19 were ascertained. It was clear by the nature of the virus that all of humanity would ideally need to be vaccinated to prevent mutations as well as the spread of the virus. There was a realization that no one was going to be safe until everyone was safe—a phrase attributed to Mark Lowcock, who served as the UN under-secretary-general for humanitarian affairs and emergency relief coordinator.[14]

The odds were stacked against the quick development as well as against rapid global scaling of any vaccination programme. Historical precedents showed that a quick turnaround for a vaccine had several hurdles. Vaccines contain small fragments of the very organism that causes the disease the vaccine is supposed to blunt. They also need substances like adjuvants, diluents, preservatives, residuals, stabilizers and surfactants to create the correct, medically effective combination that does its job.[15]

Given the complexity of the research and development effort behind creating a potential vaccine candidate, the initial work on vaccines has been traditionally done by universities and research laboratories. The pharmaceutical companies may not always take the first stab at the research and development process, given the financial and operational risks and the potentially long timelines.

Once the pharmaceutical companies get involved, they lead the process to take the vaccine to the market after due regulatory procedure. The vaccine candidates undergo multiphase trials to demonstrate not just the effectiveness but also the safety of the vaccine. Humongous quantities of data are collected through these human trials, which are then reviewed by the designated medical and drugs authorities in the country where the vaccine is intended to be launched.

The long-drawn process of researching, testing and making vaccines fit for human use means that their availability and mass deployment have lagged behind. A look at the viral pathogens identified in the last century is instructive and captures the challenge the world faced at the onset of the Covid-19 pandemic. *The Vaccine Book*, published in 2016, succinctly described this uphill battle.[16]

The Yellow Fever virus was discovered in 1900. It took 35 years for its vaccine to become available.

Polio was discovered in 1909, and its first vaccine was developed for human use in 1954. In India alone, tens of thousands of children got affected by polio, leading to severe impacts like paralysis and death.

Measles was discovered in 1911, and its first vaccine was licensed for public use in 1963.[17]

The influenza virus was discovered in 1933 and its first vaccine was available in the market in 1945. In the US alone, influenza still kills between 12,000 to 52,000 individuals every year as per a study by the Centers for Disease Control and Prevention (CDC).[18]

Hepatitis B was discovered in 1967, its vaccine was put into use in 1984. Hepatitis A, discovered in 1973, had a vaccine developed for it 22 years later, in 1995.

The rotavirus, discovered in 1973, took 25 years to be countered by a vaccine in 1998.

Finally, the human papilloma virus or the HPV, discovered in 1974, was the last to get a vaccine, only in 2007, 33 years after its discovery.

In early 1963, Dr Maurice Hilleman was woken up one night by his crying, five-year-old daughter, who was complaining of a sore throat.[19] Hilleman, a microbiologist working at the American pharmaceutical giant Merck, identified her illness as mumps. He drove back to his workplace to fetch sampling equipment, swabbed cell cultures from his daughter's throat and went to work. Four years thereafter, the mumps vaccine—a live attenuated viral vaccine—was in production.

This was the fastest a vaccine had gone from initial development to production.

Hilleman's team at Merck was prolific, developing 40 vaccines over the decades, including ones for Japanese encephalitis, measles, mumps, rubella, hepatitis B and chickenpox. The Jeryl Lynn strain—named after Hilleman's daughter—is still in use in the measles-mumps-rubella (MMR) vaccine.

But throughout the spread of viral diseases, there was never an expectation that a vaccine may be invented while the virus was at its peak destruction to tame its impact, if not the spread. This possibility had never been attempted in human history. Four years is what the world had as the best evidence for the development of a successful, modern, well-tested, well-proven and globally used MMR vaccine. The world could not afford to wait for four years in the case of Covid-19 for there would not be much left to save.

The difficulties and practical problems in devising a vaccine against viral pathogens are not just demonstrated by the decades that elapse in the process; the difficulties are actually better exemplified by the fact that no vaccine has actually ever been developed for several viruses, some of which have been known to humankind for three decades to a century now.

The herpes simplex virus (HSV), discovered in 1919, the respiratory syncytial virus (RSV), discovered in 1956, and the dengue virus, discovered in 1960, have all gone without a vaccine. Dengue has become a frequently occurring disease in India every year—newspapers are flooded with stories of the debilitating, mosquito-borne disease. So, in the case of Covid-19, the question was not only whether a vaccine could be developed quickly enough, but whether it could be developed at all.

A Less-Than-Desirable Success Rate

There has been an anecdotal argument that viruses that did not impact the resource-rich western world never got enough attention for vaccine research and development. But, even in the case of the HIV, recognized as a true global health issue since 1983, a vaccine has not been devised. Similarly, the hepatitis C virus (HCV), which is the cause of some cancers, such as liver cancer and lymphomas, does not have a vaccine despite being known since 1989.

The success stories have been few and far between. To take a recent example, the first human infection of swine flu or the new influenza A H1N1 virus came to light on 15 April 2009. In a week, there were announcements of efforts regarding vaccine research. The Food and Drug Administration (FDA) approved four vaccines on 15 September of the same year. However, the vaccines were not easily available for use till several months even then. Eventually, the virus itself lost potency and did not lead to a pandemic at the scale of Covid-19.[20]

Only two infectious diseases are considered to have been successfully eradicated—smallpox and bovine rinderpest.

Smallpox, the vaccination against which began with Edward Jenner's efforts in 1796, was eradicated in 1980. The last known case of transmission was recorded in Somalia in 1977. The WHO announced its eradication on 8 May 1980.[21] In its edition dated

9 May 1980, *The New York Times* reported, 'Health ministers of 145 countries joined today in marking what is believed to be science's total victory over smallpox.'[22]

Rinderpest, also known as cattle plague, was declared eradicated in 2011. The United Nations Food and Agriculture Organization had been tracking the disease and felt confident enough to claim total eradication in October 2010.[23] The formal announcement by UN came on 27 June 2011.[24]

Global Vaccine Efforts

These were the insurmountable odds against which the first announcement towards making a vaccine to tackle Covid-19 was made. Massachusetts-based biotechnology company Moderna, one of the three partners of CEPI, was the first to announce work on accelerated development of a messenger RNA (mRNA)-based vaccine against the novel coronavirus.[25]

Jennifer Haller became the first volunteer to be administered the experimental Moderna vaccine at the Kaiser Permanente Washington Health Research Institute in Seattle on 16 March 2020. This was part of the first 45-volunteer trial in Seattle. Moderna went from sequencing the virus' genetic information to shipping a vaccine candidate in six weeks.[26]

In the United Kingdom (UK), the University of Oxford had announced research on Covid-19 vaccination efforts on 7 February 2020. However, the university intended to produce 1,000 doses of vaccines for testing and trials and, at that stage, the question of commercialization was not centre stage.[27]

Following these initial developments, *Bloomberg* broke the news of the US pursuing 'Operation Warp Speed' on 29 April 2020.[28] The American government envisaged a programme along the lines of the Manhattan Project, which produced the first nuclear weapon during the Second World War.

The administration, led by President Donald Trump, sought

to bring together private pharmaceutical companies, government agencies and military research facilities to kick-start a vaccine development effort, aiming to make vaccines available by January 2021. The programme was formally announced on 15 May 2020, a fortnight after *Bloomberg* broke the news.[29]

The American government's effort was widely criticized in the mainstream media. An article in *Bloomberg* noted: 'President Donald Trump's top medical advisers, led by the infectious disease expert Anthony Fauci, have repeatedly said that a coronavirus vaccine won't be ready for 12 to 18 months at best.'[30]

The *New York Times* was more forceful in its criticism of the rushed vaccine development effort. One of its article read: 'President Trump is pressing his health officials to pursue a crash development programme for a coronavirus vaccine that could be widely distributed by the beginning of next year, despite widespread skepticism that such an effort could succeed and considerable concern about the implications for safety.'[31]

Spotlight on mRNA Vaccines

It is pertinent to ask why there was so much global focus on the mRNA technology as the means to a successful vaccine. While the research in this field had been conducted for a long time, there had been no clear breakthrough readily available to demonstrate that the mRNA platform would deliver results on a massive scale globally.

Easier alternatives, such as the vaccines that are made through microbial fermentation technology, similar to the one used to make the recombinant hepatitis B vaccine, had been available throughout the world and had been reasonably successful. These vaccines traditionally had a good safety profile, were easy to scale up and had the lowest cost of all vaccine technologies. Yet, large pharmaceutical players did not choose these types of vaccines as their first option.

Operation Warp Speed, the most significant global investment in research and development, also focussed on innovation. The firms that were working on more traditional technologies were not part of this funding programme in a big way. The programme naturally tilted towards the primacy of new research and making it successful. One possible way to look at this decision is that the US government may have wanted to spur biotechnology research and development, without analysing the problem in terms of vaccine equity or access. While Operation Warp Speed intended to achieve a breakthrough on vaccines, its scale may have also been designed to serve as a fiscal boost to the economy. Governments around the world were considering implementing fiscal measures to address the pandemic-impacted economic downturn.

Even the CEPI did not fund other technologies in a big way. The Baylor College of Medicine in Texas, for example, received a grant from this coalition for what would become Corbevax—a successful vaccine based on an open-source technology that was used in India extensively. But this grant was less than 2 per cent of the one that the mRNA vaccine ecosystem received.[32]

The CEPI also released an early guideline that certain types of adjuvants—the substance which enhances the human body's immune response to an antigen—were not fit for use in Covid-19 vaccines. Policies that discouraged using aluminium-based adjuvants would make it difficult for developing countries to think about vaccines, as these were the most commonly used adjuvants there. Hence, the initial design choices for the vaccine, which had financial backing, were already stacked against the developing countries and favoured engagement with large pharmaceutical players.[33]

It may have been quite possible that many governments and non-profit organizations did not think of Covid-19 as a true global pandemic. Perhaps, the intent was to use this health event as a platform to push the mRNA technology, which then could have been improved for a 'real' pandemic down the line. Another potential motive could have been to use the Covid-19 pandemic as a 'testing ground' for a new technology. The possibility that the entire world may need the vaccine was perhaps not an active consideration.

Unfortunately, Covid-19 proved to be a global disaster. Though there was considerable focus on mRNA vaccines, they satisfied none of the criteria making up the vaccine trilemma—equity, access and affordability. These vaccines were going to be based on a new technology, the research and development for which was happening in real time. Hence, neither the ability to make these vaccines at scale nor their price was going to suit most of the world. This would naturally impact vaccine access negatively, with too many countries and too many people chasing a slowly increasing supply of vaccines based on a new technology.

Be that as it may, the western world, especially the US, decided to partner with the pharmaceutical firms directly.

3

THE RACE TO THE FINISH

With the clear acknowledgement that modern vaccine development was a long drawn out and expensive process prone to failure, different countries took different approaches for developing their vaccines. The US decided to assume financial, operational and reputational risk with the aim of collapsing the typical time taken for development of vaccines (5 to 15 years) without worrying about the costs, which could be up to 1 billion dollars (nearly ₹8,000 crore).

The US took this path with the full understanding that there was no guarantee that the process would succeed. After all, no vaccines against viruses had been made easily or quickly.

In the western world, in general, the pandemic response was characterized by the sheer financial weight and capability they brought to bear upon vaccine and drug discovery, in addition to rapid efforts to accelerate vaccine development and trialling timelines.

All the big names got started. These included Johnson & Johnson, Merck, Pfizer, GlaxoSmithKline (GSK), Sanofi and Novartis. All of these firms had past experience in making vaccines, and many of them were involved with initiatives like Gavi to produce vaccines at a large scale.

Some of these firms leveraged in-house capabilities, while others tied up with specialized development entities. While Merck went at it alone, Johnson & Johnson turned to its wholly owned subsidiary, Janssen Pharmaceuticals. Pfizer tied up with BioNTech of Germany. GSK and Sanofi partnered with each other.

A number of smaller companies, too, started developing vaccines. The new mRNA technology for vaccines received particular interest. Moderna in the US and CureVac in Germany both proceeded down the mRNA path to develop vaccines. Others, like Janssen, took a more conventional viral vector path. Valneva—like Bharat Biotech in India with Covaxin—took the inactivated vaccine route.

TABLE 1

Operation Warp Speed: Vaccine Development Investments[1]

Company	*Type*	*Contract Value*	*Order Size*
Pfizer/ BioNTech	mRNA	$5.7 billion	300 million doses
Moderna	mRNA	$4.94 billion $954 million	300 million doses (development)*
AstraZeneca/ Oxford	Viral vector	$1.2 billion	300 million doses
Johnson & Johnson/ Janssen	Viral vector	$1 billion $456 million	100 million doses (development)
Novavax	Protein subunit	$1.6 billion	100 million doses
Sanofi/GSK	Protein subunit	$2.04 billion $30.8 million	100 million doses (development)
Merck	Viral vector	$38 million	(development)

*Development of vaccines that needed more work and resources

The US: Operation Warp Speed

These efforts were quickly backed in the West with enormous government funding. The most high profile of these was Operation Warp Speed.[2] It committed a colossal $18 billion (₹1.35 lakh crore) across multiple pharmaceutical companies and supply chain entities to accelerate the development and production of vaccines, along with orders for a total of 1.2 billion doses of vaccines.

The US aggressively pushed vaccine development efforts. It started coordinating with health agencies towards a response early on.

The National Institute of Health had a multi-year record of mRNA research collaboration with Moderna, and, in fact, the two parties were involved in a patent dispute for a long time. Moderna only backed down from this patent dispute in December 2021.[3] The foundations of such direct government–industry collaboration, with the government 'going into business itself' with the vaccine makers, were already in place.

The American view was that if a sufficiently large amount of money was thrown at the problem, ultimately private enterprise would find a way. The American sociopolitical system would accept such a proposition, where theoretically $18 billion could be spent on a process that had a low probability of success.

A similar approach may not have been accepted in most other societies. Fiscal prudence is a very socially contextual idea, and perhaps no other country would have accepted such an upfront investment.

In fact, what's not highlighted in the vaccine development process is that a lot of the American investments either failed outright or did not produce the expected returns on investment. Yet, this situation was acceptable in the US simply because the country had the necessary resources, and the concept of failure was much less taboo there than most other parts of the world, especially in the financial sense.

Europe: Catch-up Game

Meanwhile, the European Union (EU) struggled initially, acting much more slowly and less decisively than the Americans and the British in combating Covid-19. The Americans aggressively courted European pharmaceutical companies for collaboration, even as the EU was slow to do so.

On 11 February 2020, the American government agency Biomedical Advanced Research and Development Authority (BARDA) announced[4] a collaboration with Johnson & Johnson /Janssen, and a week later partnered[5] with the French firm Sanofi for potential vaccine development. In mid-March, Pfizer and BioNTech announced their partnership. At the same time, the US government reached out to the German CureVac—an mRNA vaccine pioneer—to collaboratively develop a Covid-19 vaccine.

These actions set off alarms at the EU headquarters and heralded the first instances of what would be an ugly dimension to the Covid-19 global response—vaccine nationalism.[6]

There was a sense of resentment about the American advances towards European companies. The EU member nations themselves wondered how vaccines would be shared amongst each other. In the midst of these uncertainties, Europe decided to play the catch-up game. On 16 March 2020, the EU President Ursula von der Leyen announced funding of CureVac's ill-fated effort, stating, 'I am proud that we have leading companies like CureVac in the EU. Their home is here. But their vaccines will benefit everyone, in Europe and beyond.'[7]

It was clear that major western entities were scrambling to ensure they had the first claim to any vaccine and the ability to control its supply outside their geographies.

It would be easy to moralize against such statements, but this was fundamentally the default response in such a crisis. Each country wanted to first look after their population. Of course, the original proponents of vaccine nationalism found it convenient to blame others for not helping the world at large once their needs were met.[8] But these mind games remain an integral part of global diplomacy, especially in a world where everything that can bring the world together—technology, healthcare, regulatory cooperation—can also be weaponized towards carving out specific fault lines.

The Role of the WHO

In the early months of the Covid-19 threat, the WHO's response to the growing crisis received much criticism. It waited until 30 January 2020 to declare the Covid-19 outbreak a public health emergency of international concern (PHEIC)—only the sixth time since 2005—and further until 11 March 2020 to finally declare the outbreak a pandemic.

The WHO is empowered by the International Health Regulations, a legally binding article of international law, last updated in 2005 that came into force in 2007. Signatory nations are required by law to promptly notify the WHO of disease outbreaks that may have significant risk of contagion. However, it does not define uniform standards and rigour required for reporting.

We now know that the first cases of Covid-19 were detected at the Wuhan Huanan Seafood Market in China as early as mid-November 2019. By late December 2019, the spread of the disease in the city and the subsequent lockdown made international news. Yet, the Chinese were slow to raise the alarm about the contagiousness of Covid-19 with the WHO. Hence, in turn, by the time the WHO could fully evaluate the situation and declare the disease a pandemic, the officially reported numbers globally were nearly a quarter of a million with almost 5,000 deaths.

Unfortunately, at the global level, the governments started to build pressure on the WHO. On 14 April 2020, the US formally announced[9] that it would freeze all funding to the crown jewel of international health. While no such drastic actions were taken by the EU, it was clear from its investments and outlining of its own response that it would also not let the WHO drive a coordinated global response.

On 4 May 2020, the EU played its own cards for influencing

vaccine availability for its member states. It announced a fundraiser that included the WHO, several major donors and states as parties.[10] The fundraiser yielded a commitment of $8 billion—funds meant for research, tests and vaccine development. The US did not participate. Instead, it announced Operation Warp Speed independently on 15 May 2020.

The EU announced its own vaccine investments.

TABLE 2

EU Vaccine Development Investments[11]

Company	*Type*	*Contract Value*	*Order*
AstraZeneca	Viral vector	$396 million	300 million doses
CureVac	mRNA	$266 million	100 million doses

The India Way

With a bunch of financial and operational constraints already stacked up not just against India but the developing world at large, India had tough choices to make. The Modi government has been characterized by fiscal prudence, and clearly the pandemic was not the time for reckless resource allocation. The government was cognizant of the fact that while vaccine development itself would make the real difference, the powder had to be kept dry to be able to respond to successive waves of the pandemic. Any large-scale shutdowns would eventually lead to economic disruptions and would require financial resources to backstop the potential damage to livelihoods.

PM Modi had been talking of vaccines from the very early stages of the pandemic. The topic routinely featured in his review meetings with officials of different ministries. A domestic vaccine solution was on the radar of the Prime Minister's Office (PMO) since March 2020.

The PMO asked Dr Balram Bhargava, director general of the ICMR, to explore domestic vaccine candidates.[12] Dr Bhargava stressed that the vaccine solution had to be pursued. Hence, alongside the global efforts focussed on vaccine ideas, which, by design, would have offered limited access, affordability and equity, India decided to run its own programme for vaccine development. The Indian vaccine development programme decided to keep this trilemma central to its effort.

India started to think about bringing to life credible vaccine candidates almost simultaneously with other parts of the world. The nation's foresight on the vaccine development front would go on to secure the country against the socio-economic impacts of the deadly pandemic a year later. This foresight and dogged struggle against Covid-19 make for a story of great scientific achievement and exceptional leadership in bringing the world together to conquer a common enemy.

However, despite the proactive and earnest efforts, India had to overcome the baggage of history.

4

VACCINATIONS IN INDIA: A MODERN HISTORY

India's prior large-scale vaccination efforts were at best a mixed bag of results. For example, smallpox was eradicated from the country only by the middle of the 1970s, when China eradicated smallpox by the mid-1960s, even as it went through the economic disaster of the Great Leap Forward and the Cultural Revolution. Thailand and Indonesia, both similarly warm, tropical countries, eradicated polio by the mid-1990s.[1] India took longer than Somalia, Ethiopia and essentially all of sub-Saharan Africa to eradicate polio—finally managing to do so only in 2011.[2] It was amongst the very last countries to successfully eradicate that scourge.

How can a nation that boasts of Serum Institute of India (SII), the world's largest vaccine maker, and a host of now well-known pharmaceutical and biotechnology companies have so much trouble conducting vaccinations? Why did India trail behind most of the developing eastern countries and Southeast Asia when it came to vaccinations?

A successful vaccination effort requires three things: access to vaccines, a mature national infrastructure for storage and distribution and an execution capacity to ensure that all citizens are able to get a vaccine dose. Historically, each of these have taken decades to accomplish, and they can be roughly divided into different periods.

From Independence to the late 1970s, India did not have broad access to vaccines.[3] At the time of Independence, India reported the largest number of smallpox cases in the world. Cholera, plague, tuberculosis and malaria presented major public health problems. The former US ambassador to India from 1973–76, Daniel Patrick Moynihan once asked, 'What does India export but communicable diseases?'[4] Given this situation, smallpox and polio present two divergent stories.

Smallpox Eradication in India

The Indian National Smallpox Eradication Programme (NSEP) began in 1962, following the WHO's global call for a concerted effort at eradication in 1959. The erstwhile Union of Soviet Socialist Republics (USSR) was the primary driver of the effort. At the Eleventh World Health Assembly of the WHO in 1958, Deputy Minister of Health of the Soviet Union Dr Viktor Zhdanov presented a lengthy report on successful Soviet efforts to contain smallpox, concluding, 'As regards its complete eradication throughout the world, we think that this can be achieved within the next ten years.'[5] It followed up by offering 25 million doses of vaccine to the WHO. The World Health Assembly formally passed a resolution calling for special programmes for its eradication.[6]

Early progress was slow, with the Indian government constrained for financial resources as well as access to vaccines. Among the major contributors to India's smallpox eradication efforts were the US and the USSR; the latter contributed hundreds of millions of vaccine doses.[7] Yet, by 1963, progress started being slow due to sporadic access to vaccines.

Frank Fenner et al. mentioned in their definitive account of the global effort to eradicate smallpox:

> Indeed, shortly after the [sixteenth] Health Assembly concluded [in 1963], the Director General made emergency

> appeals for vaccine for India to help to meet a projected deficit of 50–100 million doses a year. Few countries, however, had the laboratory capacity to make more than token contributions even if they were so inclined.[8]

By the first five years of the launch of the NSEP, India had performed half a billion vaccinations,[9] including first and second doses. Yet, cases continued to rise. A certain combination of factors were responsible for this rise—a mobile migrant labour population, lack of tracking, duplication or inaccuracy of vaccination records, a liquid vaccine that deteriorated in the heat as well as the painful 'rotary lancet' injection device that led to vaccine hesitancy.

A particular echo from the smallpox effort underlines why the design of a vaccine matters in terms of Indian usage. Fenner et al. in *Smallpox and Its Eradication* said: 'Until freeze-dried vaccines became available and regular assessment was made of the results of vaccination, many vaccinations, especially in tropical countries, were performed with vaccines of less than the required potency.'[10]

Large volumes of the freeze-dried vaccine were being produced in North American laboratories starting around 1967.[11] Between the late 1960s and late 1970s, the Smallpox Voluntary Fund received over 400 million vaccine doses, of which nearly 60 per cent were from the Soviet Union.[12] Though trained personnel were required for putting together injectable vaccines, in all, the latter were quite effective.

Despite smallpox no longer being an endemic disease in most parts of the industrialized world by the 1960s, its eventual eradication was driven by the ability of one or more nations to supply usable vaccines in bulk. This took several years to accomplish. Fenner et al. said, 'Most of the contributed vaccine was provided under bilateral agreements by the USSR, which donated more than 1,400 million doses from 1958 to 1979. The USA provided more than 190 million doses, primarily to the western and central African countries, also under bilateral agreements.'[13]

Increasing availability enabled countries to focus more on the mechanics of tracking outbreaks, containment and vaccination execution. Globally, smallpox eradication took half a decade to get to the point where the developing world could focus on execution rather than being primarily hampered by a lack of supply.

In 1970, a revised programme was announced by India in a collaboration with the WHO, focussing on a surveillance–containment approach in addition to vaccinating the young. This was due to two notable features of the Indian smallpox situation: seasonal mobile clusters formed by the movements of migrant labour and a very high impact on children due to malnutrition.

Organized and immensely data-driven, this effort also directly addressed social stigma against reporting of smallpox cases by introducing monetary awards.[14] An organized effort helped in tackling underreporting.

A notable side story of this effort was the mechanism used for vaccination. For a time, the NSEP persisted with the use of rotary lancets, despite the fact that they were painful and resulted in vaccine hesitancy, for the simple reason that the scar was easy to observe for recording purposes. This was in a much more primitive era, long before a platform like CoWIN came into existence.

By the start of the 1970s, India switched to the use of the much less painful bifurcated needle mechanism to administer smallpox vaccinations. This shift was accompanied by two additional necessities: the increasing access to supplies of freeze-dried vaccines, and a dramatic increase in the monitoring and tracking administrative infrastructure.

Within five years, this renewed effort would culminate in success—the last reported case of smallpox in India was in May 1975. This was a stunning success, by far the greatest contributor to the end of the global smallpox scourge, since India accounted for 60 per cent of global smallpox cases a decade prior.[15] In *Smallpox and Its Eradication*, the word 'India' is mentioned 1,913 times—the maximum number of times any country has been mentioned in the work.

The success of eradicating smallpox offered very important lessons on Indian strengths and weaknesses at tackling urgent public health problems. Even in the 1960s and 1970s, India could demonstrate the institutional capacity of state power to sweep the vast extent of the country in mission mode to combat a dangerous scourge. *If* sufficiently focussed, the executive state power was more than capable of getting things done.

The mechanics of executing the national smallpox surveillance, containment and vaccination plan cannot be underestimated. At the time, India had only a fraction of the roads, vehicles, telephones and other infrastructure that we have today. There were approximately 3 million vehicles operating nationwide in the mid-1970s, compared to over 300 million[16] at present. Yet, the final push towards smallpox eradication saw healthcare workers survey all of India's 100 million households at the time every month.[17]

This demonstrates how India could summon resources half a century ago to tackle and eliminate a scourge that vast parts of the country had fatalistically come to expect to be one of the harsh realities of their existence. Just a few years of concerted effort and smallpox was wiped out, just like that. A disease that ravaged the country for millennia just remains as a part of living memory for those Indians who are now in their fifties or older.

The smallpox success was possible due to the herculean efforts of those at the very top of the executive arm of the government, combined with access to generously donated vaccines and equipment. Despite the lack of basic healthcare facilities, transportation or infrastructure, India was able to overcome a major crisis by force of will. But this example also shows that a crisis occurring in a big way, in a short span of time and impacting all sections of the society, unlike smallpox, could not be tackled if there was a lack of systemic capabilities.

The global smallpox eradication effort resulted in efforts by the WHO to encourage all member states to craft universal immunization programmes of their own. India responded in 1978 by announcing the Expanded Programme of Immunization (EPI). However, this was restricted to urban areas only, which meant it offered nowhere close to comprehensive coverage in a country that had only 25 per cent urban population at that time.[18] In 1985, the EPI was replaced with the Universal Immunization Programme (UIP).

One of the beneficial, if much delayed, consequences of the Indian smallpox effort was the Minimum Needs Programme in the Fifth Five Year Plan (1974–79). The plan mandated a network of healthcare facilities of three kinds: sub-centres (SCs) for every 5,000 people (3,000 in tribal and hilly areas), primary healthcare centres (PHC) for every 30,000 people (20,000 in tribal and hilly areas) and community healthcare centres (CHCs) for every 100,000 people.

These goals were partially achieved 30 years later, during the Tenth Five Year Plan, when both SCs and PHCs were sufficient in number, but CHCs still lagged, with only 1 per 2 lakh people.[19] The CHCs and PHCs were at the frontline of vaccine cold storage facilities in the UIP and would go on to play an important role in the vaccine cold chain as part of Covid-19 response.

The regular UIP cold chain network begins at the seven Government Medical Storage Depots (GMSDs) located in the four major metros, along with Karnal, Hyderabad and Guwahati. From these seven locations, vaccine stocks reach the state, division and district vaccine cold stores, with the CHCs and PHCs being the final destination.

These initiatives began after the eradication of smallpox, but would take a generation to support a true universal immunization effort.

Thus, the smallpox eradication effort ultimately resulted in efforts to create a healthcare and vaccination infrastructure, which, up to that point, had been criminally delayed by decades. India did not have sufficient basic healthcare facility coverage until the late 2010s, six decades after Independence.

Similar problems to the ones faced while addressing smallpox were also to manifest themselves in the polio eradication effort. The first imported vaccines were not sufficiently effective—as determined by a landmark study at the Christian Medical College in Vellore in the mid-1960s.[20] This result was confirmed by further studies.[21] Low vaccine efficacy would only result in a temporary gain that was offset by subsequent outbreaks, which were unresponsive to the vaccine.

No Templates

While India saw success in smallpox eradication, the contemporaneous tuberculosis and polio efforts were far less successful.

India had tuberculosis vaccine production capabilities as far back as Independence. However, its eradication effort continues to the present day, a legacy of a long history of floundering pilot projects that could not be scaled up nationally as a result of the lack of political will, vaccine hesitancy, lack of production capacity and essentially a permutation or combination of these.[22] It is only in recent years that India has again started giving a concerted push to eradicate tuberculosis, keeping the year 2025 as a target for achieving this milestone.[23]

Polio was eradicated just a decade ago. The Pulse Polio Programme was one of the best known mass vaccination programmes targeting polio and was also one of India's public health successes. Yet, India was also one of the last countries to eradicate polio.

The polio vaccination depended on imported oral polio vaccines (OPVs), initially, but its efficacy against the strains prevalent in India was not high as was concluded in the mid-

1960s in a landmark study at Christian Medical College, Vellore.[24] One of the factors that impeded the Indian effort was the shift from Jonas Edward Salk's original inactivated polio vaccine (IPV) to the use of the OPV.[25]

India committed to the 1988 declaration of the World Health Assembly to eradicate polio. The Pulse Polio Programme, the official intervention India made in this regard, started in 1995. It took a little more than 16 years from that point to get the job done.

All these examples demonstrate the fine line between success and failure of a mass vaccination effort. Even the lack of critical elements like local vaccine production capability, as in the case of smallpox, can be compensated with access to generously donated supplies of effective vaccines. It does mean a long wait of several years, but backed by strong administrative support, it can work. However, the same situation, but with less than effective vaccines, as in the case of polio, dooms the effort to years or even decades of delay.

These historical references are important to note. Discussions around Covid-19 vaccines—the demands made from the government, the expectations from the medical fraternity and the problems encountered in the field—had all been seen before. These issues were quite real and had to be factored into the decision-making process.

Covid-19: Amplified Magnitude, Constrained Timelines

When Covid-19 hit, the Indian government knew what was to be done. The clear must-haves were one or more effective vaccines, the immediate ability to obtain supplies in volume and at low cost, ideally from domestic sources, leveraging the newly developed network of PHCs, CHCs and cold chain facilities, and replicating the national mission-mode effort that characterized the smallpox eradication effort, but with a more modern vaccination registration, recording and tracking mechanism.

In other words, all that was required of the Covid-19 effort was that the government target multiple simultaneous achievements that had hardly even been individually accomplished in the history of vaccination efforts in India.

What India had previously achieved over decades had to be achieved in a year, with no margin of error. The virus was dangerous, it spared no one and it could ravage societies—as we know in hindsight. Several countries have had their economies destroyed and the list of those knocking on the doors of the International Monetary Fund has become longer at an exponential pace since the pandemic.

It was critical for the Indian government to avoid making the same mistakes again. Principal among them was just access to vaccines. India had lacked the ability to either develop or produce vaccines on a self-sufficient scale in the smallpox era. India's success in tackling smallpox was contingent on the availability of imported vaccines.

The global nature and complexity of the Covid-19 pandemic meant that hope could not be a strategy. If the Indian vaccination plan was to hinge on imported vaccine supplies, it would not just be an obvious failure, it would be a non-starter. This was clear, as such a plan would have taken several years to accomplish for a simple reason: India's population. It would be fundamentally impossible to align the profit motive of a foreign producer with the contradictory need on India's part to have access to approximately one-sixth of global supply of a vaccine at the lowest possible cost.

This situation can be compared in an intuitive way to how businesses operate in India. Every Indian city has local eating joints of great repute, impeccable quality and unmatched product efficacy. Such joints run for decades, carrying the same laurels simply by word of mouth for their captive audience.

Let's say that a hypothetical joint of this nature serves the best pani puri to customers. Inspired by the reputation of this joint, the central government asks the proprietor to serve pani puri not to a few hundred customers on a given day, but to the whole country in a few months. To top it, five more countries approach the same reputed seller for pani puri to feed their population, too, in the same timeframe but keeping costs low. Could a bespoke player—reputation and track record aside—scale from a single shop to multiple countries in a few months? It would be hard to align the motives of the buyers and capabilities, willingness and abilities of the seller.

Vaccines are far more complex than pani puri. The product's success circumstantially depends on various things, not just the product itself. For example, even the mode of administration of the vaccine might require prior permissions to be cleared and occasional payments before it can be used. This occurred in the case of smallpox. A little-known fact about the eradication effort is that the bifurcated needle that enabled more effective vaccination was a patented product. Dr Benjamin Rubin from Wyeth Laboratories in Pennsylvania, US, is credited with its invention in a patent awarded in 1962. After negotiations with the WHO in the late 1960s, Wyeth agreed to waive licensing costs of the needle, but only for use in developing countries.

This is a small example of how intellectual property barriers can impact a large vaccination effort. These barriers exist not just with the actual vaccine, but even such things as the needle used. To obtain access at preferential rates requires multiple things—the ability to negotiate from a position of strength, the way WHO could for smallpox vaccine needles, and a willingness to wait because the patent holder would desire to first amortize the costs by earning royalties in higher-income regions.

For any large-scale vaccination requirement, or even in general anything that the country needs in very large quantities involving mass production, India was to be best served by leveraging its own low-cost production capability from companies who had a personal stake in the success of vaccinating the population of the country. The government understood the criticality of engaging private firms, who had the required expertise, to ensure that India was not left import-dependent for the supply of Covid-19 vaccines.

India's Recent Vaccine Development Capabilities

The Indian pharmaceutical industry began to grow on the global level in the 1970s. One key area behind the success of Indian pharmaceutical firms was making the generic versions of off-patent drugs. These generic versions could then be exported to global markets and would provide a low-cost alternative to consumers.

In the year 2020, India accounted for $17 billion in pharmaceutical exports, gaining around 4 per cent of the total $426 billion market share.[26] While there are several drug categories where India is a volume leader, the value of Indian exports places India as the world's tenth- to twelfth-largest pharmaceutical exporter in the last few years.

While the pharmaceutical success story is commendable in itself, it also shows that the industry has a long way to go in catching up with high-value product development, and their global acceptance and usage. Indian innovation has historically been focussed on process improvement and pricing, not so much on attacking new targets of drug development.

Vaccines provided an opportunity to the Indian industry to pivot to more research and development-oriented products. In the early 2000s, the Indian industry started taking the opportunity of vaccine-making for global supply seriously. However, even this effort was focussed on genomes that were known. Given the complex biological process of vaccine-making, a developing country like India could neither focus on new pathogens nor stockpile vaccines speculatively for spread of new pathogens.

However, things had started to change at the margins. Programmes such as the Atal Innovation Mission were building on this need for local innovations for local problems. Years ago, PM Lal Bahadur Shastri had given a call of '*Jai Jawan, Jai Kisan*', reflecting the national consciousness of the times. Later, PM Atal Bihari Vajpayee added '*Jai Vigyan*' to this national goal. When PM Modi assumed office, he started to focus on grassroots innovations. He stressed early on that scientific temper and innovation would be key to India's progress and expanded on the Indian ambition with his call of '*Jai Anusandhan*'.

The Indian research and development focus has been picking up through the previous decade, including that in the vaccination domain. PM Modi launched Rotavac by Bharat Biotech, the first vaccine developed under the 'Make in India' initiative in 2015.[27] Bharat Biotech also filed the first global patent for the Zika vaccine in 2016 after an outbreak in Brazil in 2015. The speed of this patent filing shocked the CDC, the regulator in the US, and Anvisa, the Brazilian Health Regulatory Agency.[28]

In parallel, the Indian vaccine-making industry got a leg up from the international buyers searching for cost-effective manufacturing solutions at scale. The industry saw greater private investments on vaccine manufacturing, especially after Gavi started sourcing these products from India.

Gavi was formed in 2000, with the Bill and Melinda Gates Foundation (BMGF) taking a lead in the effort as a successor to the Children's Vaccine Initiative, formed in 1990. It was supported by organizations like the WHO, United Nations International Childrens' Emergency Fund (UNICEF) and the World Bank. Gavi aimed to pool in vaccine demand from low- and middle-income countries, and then find vaccine suppliers who would be able to satisfy the large aggregate demand at a low price.

This was also the era when the Indian pulse polio vaccination programme was taking off in a big way. Greater awareness about vaccines was beginning to form. The UIP for children also began to take shape at the turn of the century, further boosted by the National Rural Health Mission.

Gavi also started to engage more with Indian vaccine makers in an effort to counter the monopoly of a few large western pharmaceutical companies. Armed with donations from key multilateral institutions and several governments, Gavi saw an opportunity to use low-cost vaccine makers in India as a way to both expand the supply side of the market as well as support India, one of the 73 countries that Gavi supplies vaccines to.[29]

With these developments, India saw the coming together of several catalysts in shaping a homegrown vaccine industry. The demand for vaccines was always present in India to counter the high infant and maternal mortality rates. With the global focus on sourcing large quantities of these vaccines and the commensurate availability of funds, the supply side started to develop rapidly. The Gavi-led sourcing from India became so strong that, by 2019, 60 per cent of all Gavi-produced vaccines were being manufactured in India.[30]

Gavi's experience in India had an interesting dimension. Gavi shaped a pentavalent vaccine starting 2005. The pentavalent vaccine protects children from five life-threatening diseases—diphtheria, pertussis, tetanus, hepatitis B and HIB. This vaccine was being sourced from India right from the early years of its introduction. However, the vaccine was not part of India's immunization programme for a while. A lot of hesitancy was built up through activism, involving specific hospitals and a network of lawyers. However, later the same hospitals were prescribing the pentavalent vaccine and earning huge profits while managing to stall its introduction in the mass immunization programme. India was one of the last countries among the 73 Gavi-supported ones to adopt the pentavalent vaccine, despite Indian companies being key manufacturers.[31]

In January 2016, the Gavi CEO, Dr Seth Berkley, met PM Modi in New Delhi to discuss the unique partnership Indian industry had formed with Gavi over the years. In a 30-minute meeting, the PM brought up several ideas and paid full attention to the proposals raised by Berkley.[32] Eventually, the Gavi CEO supported the development of the Electronic Vaccine Information Network (eVIN), which would go on to play a key role in India's Covid-19 vaccination programme.

Developments through the recent years had ensured that the government understood the complexity and the demands of vaccine production very well. A lot of pieces had to fit together to go from an idea of a vaccine to a jab in the arm. The government was well aware that it had a key role to play in the process at every stage. Leaving the process to the market forces would not be an option for a disease like Covid-19. This clarity in the system and PM Modi's personal engagement in this space with key global organizations ensured that India's recent capabilities in terms of vaccine development were leveraged from the get-go of Covid-19 vaccination.

Government Intervention: Market Making

India's vaccine needs were very particular—its sheer population meant a preference for low-cost high-volume suppliers. Its conditions, ranging from ambient temperatures to the available vaccine cold storage requirements, directly impacted the choice of technologies to pursue. The ability to independently develop or modify existing technology to serve these onerous requirements was a critical act of technological value addition in itself.

Small companies in this domain may not have been able to independently commit to spending for the research and development needed for such technological efforts. Here, the government can play a role—license technology developed in publicly funded central or state laboratories, coordinate public–private partnership (PPP) efforts with such companies to develop technology collaboratively and ensure their financial viability through multi-year order flow.

The government demonstrated clarity in its vaccination

strategy. Since India was a key player in the manufacturing market, there was a prerogative on the part of the government to foster their creation and ensure that their technological and manufacturing capabilities are supported with a long-term plan for engagement in the national vaccination design. There were some companies in the nascent stage of capability development, and this set of companies could potentially be engaged for boosting the research process.

Eventually, the government became the market maker in the process. It tried to engage in every step of the vaccine development in different forms.

From supplying better information, promoting private–public dialogue, directly financing research and development, assisting in clinical trials, handholding for regulatory approvals and international filings and placing advance orders with order-book visibility, the government did practically everything that was possible to meet a singular goal: attacking the Covid-19 virus through domestic capabilities and cutting off uncertainties born out of exogenous dependencies.

5

MAKING DHANVANTARI, SUSHRUTA AND CHARAKA PROUD

India's medical traditions are centuries old. The Ayurvedic system has had a significant place in the lives of Indians from time immemorial.

Lord Dhanvantari, considered an incarnation of Lord Vishnu, is prayed to as the founder of the Ayurvedic system of medicine. Dhanvantari Jayanti is celebrated as Ayurveda Day every year. Sushruta, considered the first Indian surgeon, has his statues installed from Kochi in Kerala to Melbourne in Australia. The *Charaka Samhita* written by Rishi Charaka is considered one of the three foundational texts of the Indian medicine system.

In the modern era, India has kept alive its pharmaceutical traditions by capturing the high-volume generic drug market. India was already home to large vaccine manufacturing facilities, with several companies at the forefront of the global vaccine supply. Indian companies fulfil more than 50 per cent of the total global demand for various vaccines that are required for the ongoing global immunization programmes.[1] India has been a global leader in vaccine manufacturing capacity and supplies for several years, even before Covid-19 hit the world.

But the Covid-19 vaccines presented the impossible combination of four challenges. Firstly, there was the epidemiological challenge of the virus and its structure not being well known. Secondly, there was thc pharmaceutical research constraint of the time available for the vaccine development effort being very short. Thirdly, there was the public health challenge of running the vaccination programme at a massive scale, not just in India but globally too. Finally, there was a fourth cross-cutting challenge: there was no precedent anywhere that guided how to overcome any of the other three challenges.

Not only was the world flying blind into the Covid-19 pandemic, it was also flying blind into devising the vaccination solution. Of course, the visibility kept on improving gradually on both the fronts. Rapid scientific interventions helped public health authorities around the world understand both the problem as well as the solution better. Yet, the problem was deterministic and already upon the world. The solution was illusory and in the stochastic domain.

India's vaccine development story, however, moved in lockstep through 2020 with the other countries working on similar initiatives. The SII started parallel negotiations to license two vaccines—the Oxford/AstraZeneca candidate AZD1222, later to be known as Covishield, and the Novavax candidate, NVX-Cov2373, labelled as Covovax. Bharat Biotech took the more conventional path of inactivated virus-based vaccines, getting immediate support from the ICMR and the National Institute of Virology (NIV).

Understanding the Virus

Extraordinarily, the NIV reported the first isolation of the Covid-19 strain NIV-2020-770 from viral samples in February–March 2020 itself.[2] Within weeks, Bharat Biotech had a vaccine candidate, BBV152, based on the NIV-2020-770 strain, which later developed into Covaxin.[3] Bharat Biotech relied on the government collaboration for the virus sequencing and isolation to make sure that private individuals were not put at risk in this process. The company had the capability to isolate viruses in its Biosafety

Level-3 (BSL-3) facilities. However, government intervention also set the right example for PPP.[4]

India became the fifth country after China, Japan, the US and Thailand to isolate the strain from virus samples.[5] All these countries had a significant number of the Covid-19 cases by then and had more samples to work with.

When the NIV, Pune, worked on identifying the various virus strains, India still did not have as many cases for the laboratories to work with. However, the success of the Pune-based institute was an important first step. Containing the virus outside the human body would help scientists understand the biology of the virus and its evolution.

This scientific success was important because it would help in developing drugs, vaccines and rapid diagnostic test kits, Dr Bhargava explained.[6] In March 2020, the immediate application of this process was the development of test kits. At that stage, barring the NIV, there were very few institutions capable of simply testing the throat and nasal samples.

The NIV was, of course, not new to coronaviruses, as H1NI was effectively the first novel coronavirus. The laboratory had also been at the forefront of India's fight against the swine flu epidemic a decade ago. This institution was set up in 1952, when the ICMR partnered with the Rockefeller Foundation. Originally called the Virus Research Centre, the institute was designated as a collaborating laboratory of the WHO in 1967. The Rockefeller Foundation withdrew its support the same year and since then, the institute has been functioning as the crown jewel of the ICMR in the field of virological studies. The NIV started functioning as the regional centre of the WHO for Southeast Asia for arbovirus studies from 1969. The institute got its present name in 1978, after being designated as an institution of national eminence.

Once the virus was isolated in Pune, the central government as well as various state governments stepped up their efforts to set up swab testing facilities around the country. At the start of the pandemic, samples had to be flown in to NIV, Pune, for testing. After the isolation of the virus, testing could be scaled nationally. This was a critical step for a faster response to the pandemic. This small milestone was further bolstered by scientists getting access to blood and swab samples of the infected patients.

Earlier, in March, the government had constituted an empowered committee, co-chaired by Professors Paul and VijayRaghavan. This committee was entrusted with the job of coordination amongst all science-backed resources at the country's disposal, including regulators, government and private research and development organizations, industry players and scientists. The mandate of this committee included working with the Department of Science and Technology (DST), the Department of Biotechnology (DBT), the Council of Scientific and Industrial Research (CSIR), the Defense Research and Development Organization and the Indian Institute of Science (IISc) to facilitate faster decision-making on all issues related to the pandemic.[7]

On 21 March, this empowered committee permitted scientists access to collected blood, nasal and throat samples from Covid-19-infected people. This announcement resulted in immediate interest in research projects involving the genome sequencing of the virus as well as further solidification of ideas regarding a potential vaccine.[8] PM Modi had already stressed the need for domestic vaccines in the earliest review meetings, and it was followed by immediate interest from the industry.

Different companies pursued different paths. Zydus Cadila pursued a novel DNA-based vaccine, ZyCov-D, which would go on to become the world's first successful DNA-based Covid-19 vaccine. Gennova pursued the cutting edge mRNA technology. Bharat Biotech pursued a novel nasal vaccine candidate BBV154, along with developing Covaxin.

By the end of March, more than 20 Indian institutions, spread across the public and the private sector, were already working on a potential vaccine for Covid-19.[9] From the public sector, the ICMR and the NIV were the key actors. The government had also received more than 7,000 tech-based proposals from various institutions and individuals around the country to work on various items of medical need associated with the pandemic.[10]

First Step in Fighting the Virus: Buying Time

PM Modi cancelled the Holi celebrations in early March as a signalling effort. He delivered televised addresses on 19 and 24 March explaining the risks emanating from the upcoming pandemic. His call of Janata Curfew on 22 March was well heeded by Indians, demonstrating his influence on the citizens. That the country paid attention to his words with full trust was remarkable and perhaps unique in the global context. When he appeared on the television screen for the second time to talk about a national lockdown, he repeatedly appealed for full compliance. His approach was to create 'awareness without fear'.[11]

PM Modi was also conscious of the fact that while masking was the only known way to escape the virus, there may not be enough masks in the country. In his meeting with the chief ministers (CMs) on 11 April, he was seen wearing a homemade mask,[12] in yet another effort to communicate the demands of fighting the pandemic. In fact, he used masked pictures as display pictures on his social media handles for a long time, stressing the importance of wearing masks. It is noteworthy that several countries continued to avoid masking mandates and many leaders certainly did not set personal examples well into the pandemic. This was a big difference between others countries and India.

India bought time through a series of policy measures to address the proximate health emergency. Access to new test kits, opening new laboratories to test viral swabs, capacity building in the public and private sector for such testing and increasing medical capacity on items like ventilators and oxygen equipment were the immediate priority.

Through March 2020, basic protection items, like hand sanitizers as well as good quality three-ply and N95 masks, were in short supply. The central government had to ensure that these constraints were removed first. The Ministry of Finance relaxed procurement rules for essential equipment for specific departments and ministries, namely Department of Pharmaceuticals, Department of Consumer Affairs, Ministry of Health and Family Welfare, Ministry of Textiles, and Ministry of Civil Aviation. Due to these changes, India could quickly procure more than ₹30,000 crore worth of life-saving essentials, including medicines, PPE and testing kits within a few weeks.[13]

The steps taken in March slowed down the spread of the virus, and the country's medical capacity was enhanced. The last week of March was tumultuous.

The cycle of internal movement of people started to reverse as the national lockdown came into force. Indians, who had come to urban centres of economic activity, began to return to their hometowns. This situation tested the limits of India's federal system. While some states stayed away from the 'us over them' style of decision-making when it came to providing relief to citizens, some states unfortunately othered the Indians who formed the backbone of local industries, like construction, manufacturing and farming. Migrant workers moved out of metro cities, like Bengaluru, Delhi and Mumbai, among others, and industrial centres, like Indore, Jaipur, Pune and Surat.[14] Some cities did a better job than others in supporting these workers. Unfortunately, not everyone received equal support in reaching their hometowns.

The central government also had to work on a plan to unlock the country in a phased manner as the initial three-week lockdown came to an end in mid-April. To top this off, there was widespread fear in the government machinery that, since the pandemic had spread first in the cities, any large movement of migrant workers to the hinterland would also expose villagers to the virus. Such movement of people could lead to unprecedented catastrophe, suffering and death caused by the highly contagious virus.[15] Public health authorities in April continued to focus on managing and mitigating this situation.

Multiple Threads of Government Intervention

Through this uncertainty and fear, public agencies were keeping an eye on how the research on vaccines was progressing. Indian agencies and scientists were closely coordinating with the WHO to follow the vaccine developments on the global front.[16] While the research institutions were focussed on the indigenized manufacturing of items like sanitizers, masks, PPE and ventilators, the DST continued to push the Indian efforts on vaccine research.

The Science and Engineering Research Board (SERB), an autonomous body under the DST, launched the Intensification of Research in High Priority Area (IRHPA) programme, where it invited proposals to ramp up countrywide research and development efforts in late March. These proposals included areas like epidemiological studies, immune response studies, affordable diagnostics as well as new anti-viral drugs and vaccines.[17] Additionally, the SERB also invited applications for a short-term Core Research Grant Special Call on Covid-19 on various topics, which included computational identification and validation of Covid-19 molecular targets.[18] Any breakthroughs in research on this front would help the potential vaccine makers.

Through these efforts, the SERB chose five projects to scale, which included study and development of antibodies against the receptor-binding domain of the spike glycoprotein of coronavirus.[19] This effort eventually helped understand the efficacy and effectiveness of vaccines.

Even as the national migrant crisis was unfolding, hundreds of scientists around the country had started work on yet another crucial aspect of vaccine development—genome sequencing.

The effectiveness of any vaccine is a function of the knowledge of its genome sequence. Using an inactivated or an attenuated virus, along with the knowledge of its genome sequence, is considered the most effective way to develop vaccines against viruses that are not well known.[20] Genome sequencing leads to the understanding of the genetic material found in the virus. The genomic sequence provides details at the level of deoxyribonucleic acid (DNA) segments. It can help scientists determine which stretches of DNA contain genes and which ones carry regulatory instructions, turning genes on or off.[21]

As the scientific community got together, often using virtual platforms to coordinate with each other, and as the empowered committee started bringing together the whole-of-government approach to the research efforts, the genome sequencing process took off.

Three institutes operating under the CSIR, namely the Centre for Cellular and Molecular Biology (CCMB), Hyderabad, the Institute of Genomics and Integrative Biology (IGIB), New Delhi, and the Institute of Microbial Technology (IMTech), Chandigarh, led the genome sequencing efforts. Organizations affiliated with state governments also contributed to the process. Researchers working at the Gujarat Biotechnology Research Centre also succeeded in decoding the entire genome sequence of the Covid-19 virus and identified its three mutations.[22]

Established in 1942, the CSIR is a network of 37 national laboratories, 39 outreach centres, three innovation complexes and five units across the country. It has a patent portfolio of 1,132 unique patents in force, out of which 140 have been commercialized. CSIR also has 2,587 in-force patents granted abroad in multiple countries.[23]

By early May, the IGIB, New Delhi, under the CSIR had already submitted 53 genome sequences to the Global Initiative on Sharing All Influenza Data (GISAID),[24] a Munich-based global science initiative established in 2008, which coordinates for open data collection for facilitating worldwide research on respiratory illnesses. The IGIB, set up in 1977 as the Center for Biochemical Technology, has been India's premier research institution for integrative biology.

The CSIR, led by Director General Shekhar C. Mande, also the secretary of the Department of Scientific and Industrial Research under the Ministry of Science and Technology, had yet again demonstrated why it was considered a global leader among government-affiliated research organizations, being ranked thirty-seventh among 1,587 government institutions worldwide and the only Indian organization in the top 100, according to the Scimago Institutions Rankings of 2021.[25] It also holds the seventh rank in Asia and leads the country at the first position.[26]

16 April 2020: When the Inactivated Virus Vaccine Got a Thumbs-Up

Through the various research inputs and genome sequencing information, the emerging view in the government research fraternity was that indigenous vaccine efforts should focus on the inactivated virus strategy. A crucial press release on 16 April confirmed that the decision-makers had a preference for this technology. The press release said:

> Researchers from the Centre for Cellular and Molecular Biology (CCMB) have embarked upon developing an inactivated virus vaccine for the dreaded novel coronavirus. Inactivated vaccines are known for their safety and easy production. Vaccination is thought to be the most effective and sure way to arrest the progress and deadly effect of this virus. Various organizations across the world are working towards finding a vaccine and the World Health Organization (WHO) has listed more than 42 promising candidates currently under development.

> Active virus is cultured in large numbers and then killed either by a chemical or heat. Although the pathogen is killed, or made to lose its reproduction capacity, various parts of the virus are intact. For example, the spike protein with which it enters the cells. The antigen (the chemical structure) that is recognised by the immune system is left unimpaired. When this dead microbe is introduced, the immune system is tricked to respond by producing antibodies against specific antigens still left intact, without knowing that the pathogen is dud. Inactivated polio vaccine and the rabies vaccines are made this way.
>
> As the pathogen is dead, it cannot reproduce nor cause even a mild disease. Thus, it is safe to administer to even people with lesser immunity, like the old and those who have co-morbidity.
>
> 'If we grow a large amount of virus and we can inactivate it, that will be material for candidate vaccine to be injected. Now the virus will not be active but the human body will recognise the proteins of the virus and start making antibodies against it. So, it acts as inactivated virus vaccine,' said Dr Rakesh Mishra, Director, CCMB while speaking with *India Science Wire*. Once the cell-culture-based production of the virus is in place, it would be handed over to the industry partner, he told.[27]

This press release formed a milestone for India's vaccination strategy. The clear preference within the government scientific community was to use a more predictable technology like the inactivated virus. While the production of such a vaccine would require significant precautions in using a BSL-3 facility, the administration of such a vaccine would be more predictable and easier to handle in the Indian conditions.

Research initiatives of the bodies affiliated to the DST and the DBT continued to fill various gaps required to start work for the large-scale commercial production of such a vaccine.

On 5 May 2020, the PM chaired a meeting of the task force on corona vaccine development, drug discovery, diagnosis and testing. This was the first time a formal review of the vaccine development was happening at this level. While the PM had been in the loop regarding the intermediate developments, the time was ripe for making key decisions for vaccine development.

Professors Paul and VijayRaghavan briefed the PM on the progress related to vaccine research and development. At this point, over 30 Indian vaccines were at various stages of conceptualization and research, and some were even ready to go for trials.[28] The PM instructed the members of the empowered committee to support the vaccine production process directly.

5 May 2020: Indian Vaccine Efforts Boosted

The meeting on 5 May proved to be the launch pad for India's vaccination drive. Clarity emerged from this meeting, with the PM giving clear directions on the way forward. There were three major interventions by PM Modi in this meeting.[29]

Firstly, he directed the key government officials to look at private manufacturers with existing knowledge of the vaccine-making process as partners in the final solution. He urged them to remove the distinction between the public and the private sector, and work together with a common goal of making vaccines available to all Indians as quickly as possible.

Secondly, the PM emphasized the reuse of the template deployed for the ramp-up of testing facilities, technologies and PPE kits when it came to vaccines. He stressed that the government would have to play the roles of an investor, incubator, evaluator as well as a buyer. Hence, it became very important for all arms of the government to come together and work with a common goal.

Thirdly, the PM set the tonc to fully leverage the idea of the 'the entrepreneurial state'. The government would have to bear the front-loaded risks, thus creating a backstop and cushioning for the private sector to move in with their innovation and investments. The lesson from the 2013 book *The Entrepreneurial State* by Professor Mariana Mazuccato was fully deployed by India in practice at a crucial juncture.[30]

Large, task-driven public governance systems often have context-specific characteristics and behaviours. Indian health and scientific research institutional mechanisms are no different. They are designed for long-gestation project execution at scale. The Indian central health apparatus traditionally builds the scaffolding, with the individual pieces of the buildings involving regular involvement of state governments.

The vaccine development posed a very different challenge to this institutional context. The situation required an agile and a malleable response, with a measured risk appetite. It also required functioning in a multi-stakeholder operating environment with diminished direct process control but greater time-bound outcome expectation.

Such a fundamental change requires a firm direction, clearly empowering and motivating accomplished individuals and helping them overcome hesitations. This is exactly what the PM did in the meeting on 5 May. It was clear that imagination had to drive the next steps, not the constraints.

Thus, 5 May was the tipping point.

Soon after, on 9 May, the ICMR made the seminal announcement that it was tying up with Bharat Biotech to develop a fully indigenous vaccine. India's fight against Covid-19 had turned an important corner—of being aatmanirbhar. The press release was crisply worded.

> New Delhi, May 9, 2020: Indian Council of Medical Research (ICMR) and Bharat Biotech International Limited (BBIL) have partnered to develop a fully indigenous vaccine for COVID-19 using the virus strain isolated at ICMR's

National Institute of Virology (NIV), Pune. The strain has been successfully transferred from NIV to Bharat Biotech International Ltd. (BBIL). Work on vaccine development has been initiated between the two partners. ICMR-NIV will provide continuous support to BBIL for vaccine development. ICMR and BBIL will seek fast-track approvals to expedite vaccine development, subsequent animal studies and clinical evaluation of the candidate vaccine.[31]

The Symphony of Public–Private Partnerships

A unique public-private partnership or PPP was conceptualized based on mutual trust and clear role recognition. The various arms of the government quickly and gainfully adjusted to drive an optimal outcome.

The ICMR and its affiliates narrowed down on knowing the problem better: the virus itself and its epidemiological characteristics. They also drove the process of fine-tuning the solution and conducting and supporting vaccine trials.

The institutions aligned with the Ministry of Science and Technology and the DST, like the CSIR, narrowed down on key aspects of indigenization of the vaccines. These institutions ensured that important constituents of the vaccine were domestically available.

The DBT and its affiliates jumped in to provide the necessary financial and incubation support to the private players, who were seeking to speed up research as well as trials. Biotechnology Industry Research Assistance Council (BIRAC), a Section 8 company set up under the DBT in 2012 to incubate and handhold new businesses, played the role of providing the initial capital to several vaccine candidates.

India's vaccination plan had a unique feather in its cap. Of the major pharmaceutical players that ended up developing a successful Covid-19 vaccine, India was the first to announce a PPP with well-defined contours for both sides.

The ICMR partnership with Bharat Biotech was announced on 9 May 2020. This was before the US announced Operation Warp Speed on 15 May. The UK, another major player with access to the research already conducted by the University of Oxford over the years, announced support to the industry on 17 May.[32]

The EU had been running a programme named Horizon 2020, with large financial support for vaccine development in general. This programme had been going on for several years. However, the additional funding towards Covid-19 vaccines specifically was announced only in July 2020.[33]

The one country, barring India, where government funding came in specifically for research was Australia. The Queensland government pumped in $10 million and the Australian government granted $3 million to the University of Queensland, which was part of the CEPI vaccine programme.[34] Unfortunately, this vaccine did not see the light of the day and the programme was shelved towards the end of 2020.

This analysis does not account for the plans China had for vaccines. The uncertainty around Chinese policies and the public–private interactions make it difficult for an independent judgement to be made, especially on a subject that fuelled global uncertainty.

Hyderabad and Pune: The Deccan Duo Leads

Meanwhile, as Hyderabad-based Bharat Biotech got into the thick of action, the Pune-based SII was also exploring options to enter the Covid-19 vaccine manufacturing ecosystem. This was a no-brainer for SII, which is the largest vaccine manufacturer in the world. The vaccines made by the SII were already reaching 65 per cent of all children around the world.[35] With such massive manufacturing capacities at its disposal, the company had an edge in partnering with potential vaccine license holders.

The SII approached AstraZeneca for a potential partnership. On its part, AstraZeneca had announced an agreement with the University of Oxford just days earlier, on 30 April.

The AstraZeneca press release read:

> AstraZeneca and the University of Oxford today announced an agreement for the global development and distribution of the University's potential recombinant adenovirus vaccine aimed at preventing COVID-19 infection from SARS-CoV-2. The collaboration aims to bring to patients the potential vaccine known as ChAdOx1 nCoV-19, being developed by the Jenner Institute and Oxford Vaccine Group, at the University of Oxford. Under the agreement, AstraZeneca would be responsible for development and worldwide manufacturing and distribution of the vaccine.[36]

The talks between SII and AstraZeneca ran for most part of April and May. The government itself was interested in how this discussion would progress. Prof. VijayRaghavan had been in touch with SII regularly to check on the evolution of the partnership.[37] The necessary approvals for such a partnership came through at a rapid pace in the month of May. The world knew that a true public immunization solution to Covid-19 had to go through the SII.

With secular global buoyancy in the vaccine development process in May, otherwise ravaged by the virus world over, SII was able to get into a contract manufacturing agreement with AstraZeneca very quickly. AstraZeneca agreed to manufacture 1 billion vaccine doses with SII—400 million were to be delivered in 2020.

This press release by AstraZeneca read:

> AstraZeneca has taken the next steps in its commitment to broad and equitable global access to the University of Oxford's potential COVID-19 vaccine, AZD1222, following landmark agreements with the Coalition for Epidemic

> Preparedness Innovations (CEPI), Gavi the Vaccine Alliance, and the Serum Institute of India (SII).[38]

Meanwhile, in May itself, many more Indian firms announced public plans for their own vaccine development on different platforms. In a press release, the WHO included Ahmedabad-based Zydus Cadila, Hyderabad-based companies Biological E and Indian Immunologicals as well as Bengaluru-based Mynvax, in addition to the SII and Bharat Biotech, in the list of companies that were involved in vaccine development.[39]

Swadeshi Vaccine: Sine Qua Non

By June 2020, it was clear within the government circles that domestic capabilities to manufacture vaccines were critical.[40] As the Covid-19 vaccine research progressed, it became increasingly clear that irrespective of where the virus was, the vaccines would only go where the money was.

The potential vaccine candidates emerging from the US and Europe were not necessarily going to be helpful for the Indian market. The potential vaccines were not going to be trialled in India, were likely to be costly and there would be no control over their supply, with multiple governments competing to corner their share of the vaccines.[41] It was also clear that 'moral obligations' of the producer would mean that the inhabitants of the country where the vaccine-maker was based would get prioritized in terms of vaccine supplies.[42]

While the government continued to keep all options open at this stage, the key individuals in various ministries and those advising the PM were increasingly clear in their mind that an Indian solution was going to be a sine qua non.[43]

'[…] to make India a global leader, there should be concerted efforts to activate the triple-helix model of innovation that involves intensifying collaboration between research institutes, industry, and the government,' Dr Bhargava wrote in an article.[44]

The Department of Health Research and the ICMR actively assisted all domestic vaccine manufacturers to accelerate their vaccine development process.[45]

The ICMR provided ₹10 crore assistance to the SII for conducting the trial of what would come to be known as the live attenuated recombinant vaccine Covishield. Much later, another ₹10 crore was extended to the SII for Covavax.

The ICMR extended assistance of ₹30 crore to undertake preclinical trials for the inactivated virus vaccine of Bharat Biotech, which would come to be known as Covaxin.[46] Finally, Zydus Cadila also received financial assistance for conducting preclinical animal trials for their DNA-based Covid-19 vaccine.

The DBT supported nearly 15 vaccine candidates through BIRAC. Fifteen firms such as this received more than ₹100 crore in funding for financial and technical support. The activities covered stages ranging from preclinical to clinical trials. The beneficiaries included the DNA-based vaccine of Zydus Cadila, the mRNA-based vaccine from Gennova Pharmaceuticals, Pune, the protein subunit-based vaccine of Biological E and the nasal vaccine of Bharat Biotech.

The Exhortation for an Aatmanirbhar Bharat

Aatmanirbhar Bharat has become the virtual raison d'être of the government in the post-pandemic era. PM Modi first talked about the concept on 12 May 2020 in a televised address to the nation.

The first wave of the pandemic was yet to recede then, but the country had to start opening up to contain the economic damage from the virus. As a calibrated opening of the economy was undertaken, the government introduced an ambitious and future-defining idea of Aatmanirbhar Bharat. In his address to the nation, the PM said:

If we are determined then we can reach our goals and no path will be difficult. And today there is a will and there is a way. This is to make India self-reliant. Our combined resolve is so strong that India can become self-sufficient.

Friends, this magnificent building of self-reliant India will stand on five Pillars.

First Pillar is the Economy, an economy that brings Quantum Jump rather than Incremental change.

Second Pillar is Infrastructure, an infrastructure that became the identity of modern India. Third Pillar is our System. A system that is based on the technology driven systems which fulfill the dreams of the 21st century and not the policies of the past century. Fourth Pillar is our Demography. Our Vibrant Demography is our strength in the world's largest democracy, our source of energy for self-reliant India. The fifth pillar is Demand. The cycle of demand and supply chain in our economy is the strength that needs to be harnessed to its full potential. In order to increase demand in the country and to meet this demand, every stake-holder in our supply chain needs to be empowered. We will strengthen our supply chain, our supply system built up with the smell of the soil and the sweat of our labourers.

Friends, amidst the Corona crisis, I am announcing today a special economic package with a new resolution. This economic package will serve as an important link in the 'Atma Nirbhar Bharat Abhiyan (Self Reliant India Campaign).[47]

While the country absorbed the philosophy of Aatmanirbhar Bharat, the idea was already shaping up rapidly when it came to Covid-19 vaccines. Several vaccine candidates were undergoing clinical trials at various stages. Once the local and international partnerships had been formed, the pharmaceutical firms got to work, supported by the government agencies for preclinical work and later for clinical trials.

On 15 July, nine weeks after signing the agreement with the ICMR, Bharat Biotech announced that its homegrown vaccine, Covaxin, was ready for human trials. This pace was no different from what other vaccine candidates had seen around the world. Its press release read:

> Bharat Biotech has successfully developed COVAXIN™, India's 1st vaccine candidate for COVID-19, in collaboration with the Indian Council of Medical Research (ICMR) - National Institute of Virology (NIV). The SARS-CoV-2 strain was isolated in NIV, Pune and transferred to Bharat Biotech. The indigenous, inactivated vaccine developed and manufactured in Bharat Biotech's BSL-3 (Biosafety Level 3) High Containment facility located in Genome Valley, Hyderabad, India.
>
> The Drug Controller General of India - CDSCO, Ministry of Health & Family Welfare granted permission to initiate Phase I & II human clinical trials after the company submitted results generated from preclinical studies, demonstrating safety and immune response. Human clinical trials are scheduled to start across India in July 2020.[48]

The ICMR got into a small controversy at the beginning of July. One of its statements suggested that India was going to be ready with a vaccine for public use by 15 August.[49] This supposed plan was decried and criticized by the scientific community in India and elsewhere. The media was quick to accuse the ICMR of recklessness.[50] The institution had to clarify immediately that its internal communication to Bharat Biotech was only meant to expedite the trials of the vaccine and that there were no specific plans to launch the vaccine on Independence Day.[51]

July 2020: The Balance of the Narrative Shifts

The despondency of the first wave of Covid-19, which had a long tail in India, with significant effects lasting well into September, was followed by optimism regarding the vaccines. Starting July, the balance of the conversation in India's public sphere started shifting from the disease to the potential cure.

The government also made a conscious effort to catalyse this shift. However, the government was conscious about letting the scientific community carry the more technical and substantive messages. The political class talked largely about the optimism of the vaccines itself, rather than getting into specific details on extent and limitations of vaccine effectiveness. It was important for the government to prepare the country for the idea of vaccination, rather than getting into every small detail right at the outset.

On 27 July, the ICMR inaugurated three high-volume Covid-19 test facilities to ensure that testing throughput could be sustained in the regions where the laboratories were located. The PM himself inaugurated these facilities. Speaking on the occasion, he remarked, 'Friends, talented scientists of our country are working vigorously for the corona vaccine. But till the time an effective medicine or vaccine is invented, we must wear masks and follow social distancing of "*do gaz doori*" and hand sanitization.'[52]

Speaking from the ramparts of the Red Fort in New Delhi on India's Independence Day, PM Modi included an update for the country on vaccine development. He said:

> My dear countrymen, there is a curiosity among everybody when the Corona vaccine will be ready. This is natural. This anxiety is there in everybody and everywhere in the world.
>
> I would like to tell my countrymen that our scientists are dutifully engaged in the laboratories. They are putting in great efforts. At present, testing for three vaccines is in different stages in the country. Once we get a green signal

> from our scientists, we will launch massive production of the vaccine. We have made all the preparations. We have drawn an outline to ramp up the production of the vaccines and to make it available to each and every person in the shortest possible time.[53]

This regular signposting was critical for building vaccine acceptance. This had to be done well in advance of the actual launch of the public immunization programme. The government had anticipated not just vaccine hesitancy, but also malicious campaigns against the vaccines and the immunization programmes.

The three vaccines the PM referred to in his Independence Day speech were Covaxin, Covishield and ZyCoV-D.

Clinical Trials for Vaccine Candidates

With early vaccine candidates shaping up, the next step was the critical multiple-stage trial process; it was to validate whether a vaccine is safe, efficacious and what are the side effects, if any. This leads to an immediate question—how can trials be effectively organized and funded?

Typically, the sponsor of a trial—the drugmakers themselves, usually—pays all clinical research and trial costs. Not only are clinical trials costly, they also depend on an effectively selected pool of candidates. They can be conducted independently in normal times but require careful management when multiple companies want to test their vaccine candidates: a single person cannot be given multiple vaccines due to lack of coordination and other reasons.

Western nations spectacularly announced large upfront payments to vaccine manufacturers for development and trials. India did not. Rather than handing huge sums of money to vaccine manufacturers, as western governments did, the Indian government focussed someplace else—to the DBT and the ICMR—on enable itself to activate and prepare a nationwide network of facilities for rapid clinical trials.

Nationwide, this consisted of a total of 53 sites, of which 35 were hospitals. Seven of these sites were new. They were supported by four laboratories: Dr Dang's Lab in New Delhi, THSTI in Faridabad, Interactive Research School for Health Affairs in Pune and Syngene in Bengaluru.[54] These sites collectively recruited over 1 lakh healthy volunteers for clinical trials.

This act of preparedness would have far-reaching consequences. The Drug Controller General of India (DCGI) cleared Covaxin's Phase I human clinical trials starting July 2020, which was just weeks behind heavily funded western candidates of Pfizer/BioNTech, Moderna and AstraZeneca. Covaxin would go to complete Phase II trials before the Chinese managed to get Sinovac's CoronaVac vaccine candidate past the same milestone.

Clinical trials of vaccines are expensive, with some vaccines costing upwards of $200 million,[55] or about ₹2,250 crore, to get through multiphase clinical trials. They are also time-consuming; volunteers for each phase are separately recruited. It takes months to find so many volunteers, organize them into cohorts, and even find target subgroups, such as particular age groups or health profiles.

In an act of extraordinary foresight, the government focussed on funding a national infrastructure for accelerated clinical trial implementation ahead of time. By doing so, it materially saved several months, which it would have otherwise taken had the vaccine makers been left to fund and coordinate trials themselves.

In retrospect, India correctly identified that the primary hurdle was not money but the need to domestically coordinate and unblock development or production paths as quickly as possible.

The DCGI permitted the Bharat Biotech and the Zydus Cadila vaccines to initiate Phase I and II human clinical trials. These vaccine candidates had previously undergone successful toxicity studies on rats, mice and rabbits. After reviewing this data, the DCGI permitted human trials. These trials started with 1,000 volunteers from across the country.[56]

Meanwhile, the SII also applied for the Phase II and Phase III trials for Covishield towards the end of July. The SII planned to rope in 1,600 volunteers around the country for its planned observer-blind, randomized control trials.[57]

Through this exciting yet uncertain period, the government agencies and the private firms were working in complete unison. There was no distinction between day or night, weekday or weekend. The all-hands-on-the-deck approach was visible, with all stakeholders solely focussing on getting vaccines to the market as quickly as possible after due clinical testing.[58] A wonderful example was set by this unprecedented cooperation on how the Covishield trials were approved in India.

The Phase I, II and III trials for the AstraZeneca vaccines were already on at this stage in the UK, Brazil and South Africa, witnessing varying degrees of progress.[59] The regulatory response in India was agile and factored in the already available knowledge about the vaccine.

On 22 July, Adar Poonawalla talked about the intent of submitting an application for human trials. 'We are making this application within the next 48 hours to the Drug Controller General of India's office. They will probably take about 1-2 weeks on what kind of study and trial we will have to do,' Poonawalla said, speaking to CNBC TV18.[60]

Keeping his word, the application for the trials to the DCGI was submitted on 24 July and it was reported in the media the next day.[61] Poonawalla had factored in a couple of weeks for approvals and further discussions with the regulatory authorities.

A rapid regulatory response kicked in. Firstly, the expert panel at the Central Drugs Standard Control Organization (CDSCO) took into account the data generated on the vaccine candidate during the first two phases of the University of Oxford trial.[62]

This reduced the burden on SII to start the preclinical studies from scratch and cut short the trial timeline in India.

The Subject Expert Committee (SEC) of the CDSCO then reviewed the application working over the weekend. By 28 July, the SEC gave specific feedback to the SII. While some additional information was sought, the committee also asked the SII to expand the geographic scope of the trial from the originally planned Mumbai–Pune cluster and increase the number of the volunteers.[63]

On its part, the SII responded at an electric pace. On 29 July, it submitted a revised proposal to expand the 1,600-volunteer trial to 20 selected cities around the country.[64] These sites were to include All India Institute of Medical Sciences (AIIMS), Delhi, B.J. Medical College and Civil Hospital, Pune, Rajendra Memorial Research Institute of Medical Sciences, Patna, Post Graduate Institute of Medical Education and Research, Chandigarh, AIIMS, Jodhpur, Nehru Hospital, Gorakhpur, Andhra Medical College, Visakhapatnam, and JSS Academy of Higher Education and Research, Mysore.[65]

The SEC deliberated the modified proposal, factored in the preclinical tests already done in other geographies and, by 31 July, recommended granting permission for Phase II and III clinical trials for Covishield in healthy adults in India.[66] In turn, V.G. Somani, the DCGI, sealed the approval process on Sunday, 2 August.[67]

Indian regulators and India's leading contract manufacturer of vaccines had worked together to get the clinical trial for Covishield designed and approved in 10 calendar days from the point of application. The process even included one major revision to the design of the trials. This kind of pace of work, mutual trust and coordination had been unheard of in the Indian pharmaceutical industry.

Light at the End of the Tunnel

The trials for all the three vaccines progressed at a rapid pace. As the impact of the first wave of Covid-19 started to stabilize, if not recede, a wave of optimism started to take over India's vaccine-making landscape.

The New York Times, which otherwise specialized in finding faults with everything that happens in India, profiled the SII's pathbreaking work.[68] It credited the Poonawallas for betting on a yet-unproven vaccine, investing their own money to create stockpiles in anticipation of global approvals.

Novavax, an American firm, which had a contract manufacturing arrangement with the SII, also announced its plans to bring its vaccine to the Indian market, in addition to Japan and some low-income countries.[69]

A tripartite agreement was signed between Gavi, the BMGF and the SII to produce up to 100 million doses of Covishield for low- and middle-income countries. Through this arrangement, the SII got access to $150-million funding.[70]

The Russian government authorities involved with the production of Sputnik V vaccine also expressed their interest in selecting India as the destination to scale up the production of their vaccines. The Russian authorities started the search for the Indian partners, just as Sputnik V got closer to being certified and ready for use.[71]

As science progressed, the government also started moving the wheels of diplomacy. The Indian government realized very early on that not only was there a need to make the world safer through vaccine access, but vaccine equity and affordability were also opportunities for India to stand with the countries that may not have the best resources otherwise to access the limited and hotly contested global pool of vaccines.[72]

Indian diplomats started work on five different models in which the 'Made in India' Covid-19 vaccines could be made available to various countries around the world.[73]

The first model was meant for a restricted number of immediate neighbours, such as Afghanistan, Bangladesh and South Asian Association for Regional Cooperation (SAARC) countries, excluding Pakistan. The second model was meant to cover India's international obligations, where heavily subsidized vaccines would be distributed to poor countries. The third model was that of assuring supplies of vaccines at market price. The availability itself was a premium offering, given that vaccines were not going to be sold freely in the open market. The fourth model was to enrol some countries in the Phase III trials of the two Indian vaccines—Bharat Biotech's Covaxin and Zydus Cadila's ZyCov-D. In turn, these countries could be granted preferential access to vaccines in one of the three models mentioned above. The fifth model was meant to explore coproduction of these two vaccines to expand the supply base and hence the availability.

In fact, PM Modi made a public commitment to help other countries through India's vaccine manufacturing capacity.[74] India was not just taking giant strides to protect its own citizens, the well-being of the world was also very much a policy consideration in New Delhi.

At no stage did India compromise with the quality and standard of vaccine development. In fact, Indian guidelines for the acceptance the Covid-19 vaccine candidates for medical use mirrored[75] of what the WHO had prescribed. The US had similar guidelines.

Finishing Line in Sight

The uphill climb to deploy Covid-19 vaccines against the virus finally had the summit in sight. The collective perseverance of the country and the undaunted spirit of its medical fraternity backed by an agile government response had come together in a manner never witnessed before.

Not only did the pandemic change the way countries and societies conducted themselves, it also shook the very foundation of the rules-based international order created after the Second World War. Every country had to think of its own place in the global order and ensure that it possessed the right leadership, institutional mechanisms and human capital to respond to this pandemic and whatever else may hit the world in the future. It was clear that a response to this pandemic was going to set the tone and template for any future global crisis as well. And hence, the response was not an isolated event. It was laying the foundations of new governmental, administrative and social structures.

India was up to the task of this global arranging of deckchairs. PM Modi's exhortation of Aatmanirbhar Bharat was a destiny-defining event and will remain so in the decades to come.

The public vision and private capability got together so seamlessly, especially at a time when individual suffering and unpredictability of life were at an epochal high, that they demonstrated India's true doggedness. The self-confidence built by the vaccine development process was yet another marker in India's journey to claim a greater global share of influence and voice.

But democracies seldom talk in unison, not even when it comes to celebrating a nation's own homegrown achievements. On the one hand, the government and pharmaceutical industry were moving towards a critical milestone, which would bring a sense of finality to the fight against Covid-19. On the other, a wave of disinformation, distrust and disingenuous self-loathing was about to descend on India's national discourse.

Trial and Lots of Error

Multiple vaccine candidates failed to complete their Phase III trials satisfactorily in the first attempt. In fact, the Covid-19 vaccine tracker site reported the following statistics as of September 2022, reporting about 230 candidates, including the 12 that were no longer making progress:

TABLE 3

Covid-19 Vaccine Pipeline[76]

Total Covid-19 Vaccine Candidates in Pipeline	*In Phase I*	*In Phase II*	*In Phase III*	*Approved*	*Total*
230	58	71	89	47	277

Put another way:

TABLE 4

Percentage of Total Covid-19 Vaccine Candidates that Cleared Each Trial Stage (in per cent)

Phase I	*Phase II*	*Phase III*
79	49	17

This global data shows that less than one in five vaccine candidates reached the approval stage. Barely over a third of them even cleared Phase II, meaning that they demonstrated significant antibody response, warranting a Phase III trial.

As of 3 January 2021, India had three vaccines past this critical point. Covishield and Covaxin had already received emergency use authorization that day, with ZyCov-D receiving clearance to begin Phase III trials. It is enormously significant that in a global race, where only a third of the candidates made the final step and under one-fifth of the candidates cleared all steps, India had three vaccine candidates, of which two had cleared all steps and the third cleared the critical second step.

This was the first visible measure of likelihood of national success—in a global race where major vaccine makers like Merck, Sanofi-GSK and Curevac all failed, India had multiple domestic candidates that demonstrated early success at clearing critical vaccine trial stages.

Historical data on vaccine research and development indicates that the probability of success was closer to the international data, but Indian firms had better success. Prior vaccination efforts for smallpox, tuberculosis, polio and other efforts stalled at this point—India simply couldn't acquire or produce effective vaccines. If no vaccine exists, any question of scaling up production becomes a moot point. A passable vaccine is potentially more dangerous than none at all.

Therefore, the first requirement before mass production is the demonstrated ability to develop highly effective vaccines. As early as the beginning of 2021, India had two approved vaccines with high efficacy. It had a foreign developed vaccine, Covishield, in the hands of one of the world's premier vaccine mass producers, the SII. It also had a domestic vaccine based on tried and tested inactivated vaccine technology in Covaxin. It then had the first-ever DNA-based vaccine entering Phase III trials at a time when multiple western companies, with billions of dollars of funding, had failed to get their candidates as far. ZyCov-D became the first DNA-based vaccine approved for human use. Under a dozen candidates from the US, Europe, China, South Korea and elsewhere entered the race, but ZyCov-D was the first to cross the finish line.[77]

While this may seem obvious in hindsight, the first requirement of success at producing vaccines at scale is the demonstrated ability to actually get off the starting blocks by having something to produce.

The approved vaccines were researched in the US, the UK, Germany, Russia, China and India. While some other countries were able to manufacture vaccines based on contracts, only six countries were involved in a successful research effort. A large number of technologically advanced countries with substantial pharmaceutical industries are missing from this list—France, Italy, Sweden, the Netherlands, Japan and South Korea, to name a few.

The task at hand for the Indian government was monumental. Firstly, it had to push to get hold of at least one, if not multiple effective vaccines. Secondly, it had to ensure that the vaccines could be procured at scale, ideally through local production. Thirdly, they had to be cheap, since India did not have the money to pay the approximately $25 (around ₹1,875) per dose for a minimum of two doses for a billion people, which would have amounted to $50 billion (₹3.75 lakh crore)—a sum larger than the gross state domestic product (GSDP) of half of India's states.

Although only 47 vaccines were approved globally—just one in five—not all of them saw manufacturing at scale. Just a dozen vaccines—one-fourth of those approved—started being produced in big numbers.

TABLE 5

11 Approved Covid-19 Vaccines (as of January 2021)

Country	*Vaccines/Producer*
China	EpiVacCorona, Ad5-nCov, Sinopharm BBIBP, Sinopharm Inactivated, Sinovac Coronavac
India	Covishield, Covaxin
US	Moderna, Novavax
Germany/US	Pfizer/BioNTech
UK	Oxford/Astra Zeneca
Russia	Sputnik V

Early success at producing a vaccine does not necessarily mean success at mass production. A year later, only two of the Chinese vaccines were mass produced—Sinovac and Sinopharm BBIBP. Sputnik V and the Janssen vaccines stalled after early success.

6

BEGINNING OF THE END?

'It was the best of times, it was the worst of times...'

Charles Dickens's famous opening lines from *A Tale of Two Cities* perfectly characterized the world in the fourth quarter of 2020.

The quarter was a strange combination of hope and despair around the world. Like a wound-up spring, the world wanted to bounce back from the tyranny of the lockdowns and embraced a 'just get on with it' attitude as the first wave receded. The yearning to unwind manifested itself in the hope of vaccine availability. This was visible in increased domestic travel. People were craving normalcy. The need for avoiding the virus was well understood, but the human mind wanted to be free again.

'...it was the age of wisdom, it was the age of foolishness...'

The fourth quarter of the calendar year is also the festive season around the world. India's most significant festival period from Dussehra to Diwali brings cheer and economic buoyancy every year. But in 2020, the hope remained conditional.

'...it was the epoch of belief, it was the epoch of incredulity...'

Any economic revival was predicated on early confirmation of vaccine availability. Even if the actual vaccine administration took time, society just wanted the assurance that science would eventually win over the deadly pathogen. The people in the homes and markets around India were just relieved to be able to come out in the open and celebrate Diwali. And yet, thousands of homes remained unlit in the memory of those claimed by the virus.

'…it was the season of light, it was the season of darkness…'

The trials of vaccines were progressing steadily across the globe, with different vaccine candidates seeing different levels of success. It was also becoming clear that vaccine nationalism was going to be real. The countries that would eventually have access to the vaccines would effectively be dealt a good hand in influencing global negotiations on vaccine distribution. Humankind's collective fight against the virus was the storyline. The screenplay was, however, punctuated by the dominating presence of a few key actors.

'…it was the spring of hope, it was the winter of despair'—quite literally.

Vaccines Debut in the US

The good news started to trickle in during the month of November. The chief executives of nine vaccine makers had pledged[1] in the month of September that they would abide by the rules of science and not by the rules of politics.

Put simply, the nine companies wanted to ensure that then president of the US Donald Trump did not announce any Covid-19 vaccine breakthrough before his re-election, thus separating politics from the scientific process. The nine companies were AstraZeneca, BioNTech, GSK, Johnson & Johnson, Merck, Moderna, Novavax, Pfizer and Sanofi, covering the full universe of companies likely to put out a Covid-19 vaccine in the market.[2]

They pledged to:

- Always make the safety and well-being of vaccinated individuals their top priority;
- Continue to adhere to high scientific and ethical standards regarding the conduct of clinical trials and the rigour of manufacturing processes;
- Only submit for approval or emergency use authorization

after demonstrating safety and efficacy through a Phase III clinical study that is designed and conducted to meet requirements of expert regulatory authorities such as FDA;
- Work to ensure a sufficient supply and range of vaccine options, including those suitable for global access.[3]

Each of the four statements was as much about politics and global business opportunities as about following a scientific process.

The pledge was adhered to strictly. Through the month of October and early days of November, there was regular commentary from both Pfizer and Moderna—the two firms most likely to announce a vaccine—about their respective candidates progressing well. However, material announcements, which mattered, were not made in those weeks.

On 9 November, Pfizer was first to make the big announcement. Pfizer and BioNTech introduced their vaccine candidate post successful results from the Phase III trials. The US presidential election was held on 3 November and by 7 November, it had become clear that the Democratic nominee Joe Biden had triumphed over the incumbent Republican Donald Trump.

The Pfizer press release read:

> NEW YORK & MAINZ, GERMANY--(BUSINESS WIRE)--Pfizer Inc. (NYSE: PFE) and BioNTech SE (Nasdaq: BNTX) today announced their mRNA-based vaccine candidate, BNT162b2, against SARS-CoV-2 has demonstrated evidence of efficacy against COVID-19 in participants without prior evidence of SARS-CoV-2 infection, based on the first interim efficacy analysis conducted on November 8, 2020 by an external, independent Data Monitoring Committee (DMC) from the Phase III clinical study.[4]

Moderna announced next. A week later, on 16 November, the company provided very positive data from its trials. Moderna worked on its vaccine collaborating with the researchers from the

Vaccine Research Center, part of the NIAID of the US headed by Dr Anthony S. Fauci.[5]

The UK and India Follow Suit

AstraZeneca was third. It announced good Phase III trial results from its tests in the UK and Brazil.[6] Although the efficacy of this vaccine was found to be around 70 per cent, lower than the 95 per cent figure reported by Pfizer and 94.5 per cent efficacy reported by Moderna, the AstraZeneca breakthrough was significant for several reasons. Their vaccine was easier to store and transport. The active life of the vaccine was also better managed due to its relatively less stringent storage requirements. This vaccine was expected to sell at $3 to $4 per dose[7] as opposed to the $25–$30 range per dose for Pfizer and Moderna. The Covid-19 pandemic needed not just a vaccine, but an accessible vaccine and one that could be produced at scale. The AstraZeneca product was closest to what could be a global solution.

This was also a significant breakthrough from the Indian point of view. The SII had already produced up to 40 million doses of the AstraZeneca vaccine at this stage, investing ahead of the requisite approvals. This was done at the firm's own risk after taking approvals for stockpiling.[8] If the Phase III trials failed, it would mean a loss of a minimum of ₹800 crore to SII, at an estimated ₹200 per dose, not counting all the infrastructure and related costs of establishment. With the Gavi alliance allowing SII to produce up to 200 million doses, it looked best placed to meet the global hunger for the vaccines at a reasonable price.[9]

Meanwhile, Bharat Biotech started work on its Phase III trials on 16 November. The company announced[10] a trial with more than 26,000 participants across 22 cities around the country. Not only was this designed as the largest Covid-19 vaccine trial in India, but the company claimed that this was the biggest Phase III efficacy trial to have been conducted for any vaccine before.

Bharat Biotech started at-risk manufacturing of Covaxin in late October 2020.[11] Both companies had a similar motive—to get as far ahead of the production scaling curve as they could.

The Regulatory Puzzle

The big remaining question was: when would the regulators around the world certify these vaccines as fit for the use of the general population? Despite the pronouncements on global cooperation, it was clear that regulatory arbitrage would play a key role in vaccine recognition. Not all countries were likely to accept all vaccines, even if they were approved in 'friendly' or 'partner' geographies.

Both Pfizer and Moderna filed for the emergency use authorization (EUA) for their vaccines in the US with the FDA by the end of November. The EUA in the US, as also in other countries including India, had the same purpose—if need be, the vaccines should be used as a public health requirement via programmes designed by public health agencies. However, medical professionals could not prescribe these as medicines to be bought from pharmacies. The decisions on use, methodology, stock holding as well as the actual administration of the vaccines remained with the designated health authorities.

The US FDA approved the Pfizer vaccine on 11 December.[12] The regulator made it clear that the approval process had not been completed in a hurry. It said:

> The data provided by the sponsor have met the FDA's expectations as conveyed in our June and October guidance documents. Efforts to speed vaccine development have not sacrificed scientific standards or the integrity of our vaccine evaluation process. The FDA's review process also included public and independent review from members of the agency's Vaccines and Related Biological Products

> Advisory Committee. Today's achievement is ultimately a testament to the commitment of our career scientists and physicians, who worked tirelessly to thoroughly evaluate the data and information for this vaccine.[13]

This was followed by the approval for the Moderna vaccine a week later, on 18 December.[14] Yet again, the American regulator was careful in explaining that while this was a victory of science, the approval focussed on the balance of known and potential benefits over known and potential risks. It said, 'Today's authorization demonstrates our steadfast commitment to the health of the American people, with the assurance that our scientific standards and the integrity of our review process have been maintained.'[15]

The EUA also served another purpose. There were no trade intermediaries in the business of selling vaccines. The manufacturers had full control. The governments could buy directly from the sellers and that was it. There was one set of sellers and one set of buyers, who far outnumbered the sellers. The demand was driven not just by genuine health concerns, the futures of governments were at stake, especially in democracies.

This created a huge sellers' market, which went on to more than adequately reflect in the financial performance of the key pharmaceutical companies involved in 2020 as well as in 2021. This situation put the countries with relatively high demand and less financial resources in a bind. The Indian approach for vaccine procurement was thus partly dependent on reversing this situation—using a potentially large market to tilt the balance of convenience in the buyer's favour ever so little.

The shot in the arm for India's vaccination process came with the approval of AstraZeneca's vaccine in the UK. This approval came in right at the turn of the annus horribilis. The UK Medicines and Healthcare products Regulatory Agency (MHRA) provided authorization for emergency supply of the AstraZeneca vaccine on 30 December.[16]

The press release from the company read:

> The MHRA's decision was based on independent advice from its Commission on Human Medicines following a rolling review of trial data that included an interim analysis of the Phase III programme led by the University of Oxford. The data were also published in The Lancet on 8 December 2020.
>
> Additional safety and efficacy data for the vaccine will continue to accumulate from ongoing clinical trials. AstraZeneca continues to work with regulatory authorities around the world to support their ongoing rolling reviews for emergency supply or conditional marketing authorisation during the health crisis.[17]

The press release made it clear that the UK regulator was happy with the available data. The reviews were in a 'rolling review' format, so the regulator presumably continued to engage regularly with AstraZeneca and continued to review the building evidence as it was made available. The data came from ongoing clinical trials. It was clearly established that the clinical trials were not over at this point, but the regulator was convinced that the available information was good enough for an emergency use rollout. It was a decision taken on the balance of interests again, with known benefits outweighing known risks.

The perspective of the regulators from the US and the UK is important. This sets the context for what transpired in India in the month of January 2021 and how the reactions in the popular narrative differed. The process followed by the regulators in India was exactly the same as what their American and British counterparts followed. In the UK's case, the vaccine itself was the same. And yet the Indian regulators were hauled over the coals.

The SEC of the CDSCO in India met on 1 and 2 January to review the progress of clinical trials and to review the data submitted by three firms—SII, Bharat Biotech and Zydus Cadila. On 2 January, which was a Saturday, the meeting ended with the

SEC taking a firm call on all the three vaccine candidates.

The SII was granted permission for restricted emergency use of Covishield with inbuilt regulatory conditionalities.[18] Bharat Biotech was granted restricted emergency use in clinical trial mode in public interest as an abundant precaution. Zydus Cadila was granted permission for Phase III clinical trials for its DNA-based vaccine.

These recommendations from the SEC were then ratified by the DCGI on 3 January. The press release by the DCGI was instructive and no less specific than its counterparts from the US or the UK. It said:

> The Subject Expert Committee of Central Drugs Standard Control Organization (CDSCO) met on 1st and 2nd January, 2021 and made recommendations in respect of proposal for Restricted Emergency Approval of COVID-19 virus vaccine of M/s Serum Institute of India and M/s Bharat Biotech as well as Phase III clinical trial of M/s Cadila Healthcare Ltd.
>
> The Subject Expert Committee consists of domain knowledge experts from the fields of pulmonology, immunology, microbiology, pharmacology, pediatrics, internal medicine, etc.
>
> M/s Serum Institute of India, Pune has presented a Recombinant Chimpanzee Adenovirus vector vaccine (Covishield) encoding the SARS-CoV-2 Spike (S) glycoprotein with technology transfer from AstraZeneca/the University of Oxford. The firm submitted safety, immunogenicity and efficacy data generated on 23,745 participants aged ≥ 18 years or older from overseas clinical studies. The overall vaccine efficacy was found to be 70.42%. Further, M/s Serum was granted permission to conduct Phase II/III clinical trials on 1600 participants within the country. The firm also submitted the interim safety and immunogenicity data generated from this trial

and the data was found comparable with the data from the overseas clinical studies. After detailed deliberations the Subject Expert Committee has recommended the grant of permission for restricted use in emergency situations subject to certain regulatory conditions. The clinical trial ongoing within the country by the firm will continue.

M/s Bharat Biotech has developed a Whole Virion Inactivated Coronavirus Vaccine (Covaxin) in collaboration with ICMR and NIV (Pune), from where they received the virus seed strains. This vaccine is developed on the Vero cell platform, which has a well established track record of safety and efficacy in the country & globally.

The firm has generated safety and immunogenicity data in various animal species such as mice, rats, rabbits, Syrian hamster, and also conducted challenge studies on non-human primates (Rhesus macaques) and hamsters. All this data has been shared by the firm with CDSCO. Phase I and Phase II clinical trials were conducted in approx. 800 subjects and the results have demonstrated that the vaccine is safe and provides a robust immune response. The Phase III efficacy trial was initiated in India in 25,800 volunteers and till date, ~22,500 participants have been vaccinated across the country and the vaccine has been found to be safe as per the data available till date.

The Subject Expert Committee (SEC) has reviewed the data on safety and immunogenicity of the vaccine and recommended for grant of permission for restricted use in emergency situation in public interest as an abundant precaution, in clinical trial mode, to have more options for vaccinations, especially in case of infection by mutant strains. The clinical trial ongoing within the country by the firm will continue.

M/s Cadila Healthcare Ltd., has developed a Novel Corona Virus-2019-nCov-Vaccine using DNA platform technology. The firm initiated Phase I/II clinical trials in India in more than 1000 participants which is ongoing. The interim data suggests that the vaccine is safe and immunogenic with three doses when administered intradermally. Accordingly, the firm has sought permission to conduct Phase III clinical trials in 26000 Indian participants, which has been recommended by the Subject Expert Committee.

M/s Serum and M/s Bharat Biotech vaccines have to be administered in two doses. All the three vaccines have to be stored at 2-8° C.

After adequate examination, CDSCO has decided to accept the recommendations of the Expert Committee and accordingly, vaccines of M/s Serum and M/s Bharat Biotech are being approved for restricted use in emergency situation and permission is being granted to M/s Cadila Healthcare for conduct of the Phase III clinical trial.[19]

The Regulatory Critique

The Indian regulator acted with the available data for both Covishield and Covaxin.

For Covishield, the data from AstraZeneca submitted to the British regulator was examined and found satisfactory. This data was also tallied against the immunogenicity data supplied by SII for the domestic trials. The two data sets were found equivalent in terms of vaccine efficacy. The EUA was granted with the rider that the clinical trials would continue. This stance was a mirror of the position taken by the MHRA. In fact, the Indian regulator had the added advantage of reviewing the bridge trials (the Indian trial was an additional Phase III trial, as information from Phase I and II from the AstraZeneca trial was used) conducted in India.

For Covaxin, the rolling evaluation was cited specifically. Bharat Biotech had been conducting a large Phase III trial, almost

15 times the subject size of the Covishield trial. Almost 90 per cent of the subjects in this trial had received Covaxin and the observed data was satisfactory. Hence, the EUA was granted based on a near-complete, significantly larger than usual clinical trial. The rolling data observed through the preclinical procedures as well as the Phase I and Phase II trials was found to be satisfactory in terms of vaccine safety. Also for both the vaccines, the approval was only in an emergency use mode, exactly as in the US and the UK.

India followed the same process as that followed by the developed world and, in the case of Covishield, had more data than the developed world. And yet a vituperative campaign was unleashed on India's vaccine story. Not only did the international outlets raise questions, several Indian commentators were quick to join in as well.

It is instructive to note some of this criticism, which was also factually incorrect in many cases, apart from levelling unfounded allegations.

A news report from BBC read: 'The local vaccine, however, was approved despite the absence of data on how efficient it can be. It has yet to go through large-scale trials.'[20]

The BBC was understandably charitable to Covishield, with the UK's own vaccination plan hinging on the same vaccine. But it raised doubts on Bharat Biotech's Covaxin despite the fact that the Phase III trial undertaken by Bharat Biotech was one of the largest, with 25,800-odd subjects.[21] Out of this number, 22,500 subjects had already been administered the vaccine and the SEC of CDSCO was privy to the vaccine efficacy data corresponding to these trials, as mentioned in the press release made by the DCGI.

Compare this to AstraZeneca's clinical trial, which led to the company making the application for the EUA in the UK. The AstraZeneca Phase III trial led to interim analysis of efficacy based on 11,636 participants. The safety data AstraZeneca published involved about 20,000 subjects from four trials—two in the UK and one each in Brazil and South Africa. This information was published by AstraZeneca publicly, almost a month before India's Covaxin approval.[22]

As far as Pfizer was concerned, the Phase III clinical trial, which began on 27 July, enrolled a total of 43,661 participants, of which 41,135 had received a second dose of the vaccine at the time Pfizer reported the results and used them to prepare its EUA application. The Pfizer sample was bigger, and it also ran the trial in several countries, including the US, Germany, Turkey, South Africa, Brazil and Argentina. This information was published by Pfizer on its website in mid-November.[23]

Although Pfizer did not specify[24] the division of 46,331 participants by country, the math shows quite obviously that at the most only one of the six countries could have had more than 25,000 subjects. Quite likely, no country had such a participant concentration, but even if one did, the Phase III trial of Bharat Biotech was quite comparable in size when it came to the number of individuals enrolled for clinical trials. In the press release, Pfizer also mentioned that it intended to monitor the Phase III data for two years. Thus, much like in the case of the UK, the FDA in the US also took a pragmatic view of the available data and the preponderance of evidence.

The Washington Post reported the news of Indian vaccine approval through indirect conjecture, saying:

> But the announcement was marred by questions about the fast-track approval of Covaxin, which has not completed its third phase of human clinical trials. That vaccine is being developed by Hyderabad-based Bharat Biotech in collaboration with two government-backed institutes. The regulator said the trials for the first two phases demonstrated the vaccine was safe, but it did not share efficacy data.[25]

Globally, the regulators had depended on the data submitted by the vaccine makers. This included data from ongoing trials as has been explained previously. Each regulator took a call based on scientific evidence that the data made available to them must match the expected quality and quantity to make an informed judgement on the vaccines. There was no way for the media commentators to answer that question.

However, the regulator itself was questioned, despite the fact that it was closely monitoring the vaccine development process for six months. A non-profit science journalism outlet made the following assertions: 'The approval of a vaccine without phase III data is "unconscionable" says Vineeta Bal, an immunologist at India's National Institute of Immunology.' It further added, 'Experts say such a trial is necessary because certain vaccines, such as those against polio and typhoid, have proved less immunogenic in Indians than in Western populations. But the data from SII's study have yet to be analysed fully, and the company did not respond to queries from *Science*.'[26]

In the case of Bharat Biotech, the article did acknowledge after setting the initial negative tone that, indeed, more than 22,500 participants were enrolled for the trial. Of these, the article mentioned that about 6,000 subjects had got two doses. The double-blinded trial numbers were of the same order of magnitude as the AstraZeneca trials. It would still be higher than the SII's local bridging trial.

The comment on relative geographical and ethnographic immunogenicity with respect to Covishield was again a tangential statement, more to raise quick walls of objections than to understand and critique the regulatory process.

Responding to these concerns, Dr Krishna Ella, chairman and managing director of Bharat Biotech, pointed out that the process of approval adopted in India was not unusual. In fact, the Chinese vaccine Sinopharm, also based on an inactivated virus technology, and the Russian vaccine Sputnik V were already in the market through a similar regulatory process.[27]

Indian media was not the one to be left behind either. One

article called the vaccine a political *jumla*. It read: 'Again, other than to the highly credulous, it is pretty obvious that such an "approval" was announced alongside that of the Serum Institute's Covishield for political reasons.'[28]

However, apart from making a gut-feeling-based argument, the regulators' perspective was not accounted for. The commentary was basically the tyranny of the op-ed space—the one with the access to the opinion can have a field day alleging practically anything.

For Bharat Biotech, one constraint for clinical trials was that the virus itself became less prevalent in India and even other parts of the world in the fourth quarter of 2020. The clinical trials progressed slower than anticipated. Bharat Biotech felt that there was a deliberate campaign of calumny against its product and the process. The company faced criticism from specific organizations based in India and the US, which worked on ethical issues in the pharmaceutical industry. Bharat Biotech felt that these organizations acted in tandem with select journalists to malign its image without accounting for the company's side of the story.[29]

On its part, the regulator had followed the procedures as per the applicable Drugs and Cosmetic Act, 1940, and the New Drugs and Clinical Trials (NDCT) Rules, 2019. 'Section 26B of the 1940 D&C Act gives power to the Central government to regulate or restrict the manufacture, sale or distribution of a drug by means of a notification if it is satisfied that the "drug is essential to meet the requirements of an emergency arising due to epidemic or natural calamities and that in the public interest it is necessary or expedient so to do".'[30]

The Second Schedule of the NDCT Rules, 2019, defines the process for accelerated approvals for certain drugs. Paragraph 2 of these rules addresses 'special situations for a new drug where relaxation, abbreviations, omission or deferment of data may be considered'.[31]

Paragraph 2 of the Second Schedule also identifies special situations as thus:

> For drugs intended to be used in life threatening or serious disease conditions or rare diseases and for drugs intended to be used in the diseases of special relevance to Indian scenario or unmet medical need in India, disaster or special defense use e.g. haemostatic and quick wound healing, enhancing oxygen carrying capacity, radiation safety, drugs for combating chemical, nuclear, biological infliction etc. [...][32]

This is a fairly broad definition of when drugs can be approved in special situations. It includes 'diseases of special relevance to Indian scenario', 'unmet medical needs in India' and 'disaster'. One of the questions before regulators would have been whether the Covid-19 pandemic fitted these preconditions to be called a special scenario. It would take an extraordinary mixture of bravery, cynicism and bad judgement to argue against classifying Covid-19 pandemic as a special scenario based on the above parameters.

Once it was established that the vaccines were indeed addressing a special situation, the next operative part of Paragraph 2 (ii) of the Second Schedule from the NDCT Rules, 2019, kicked in. This part said: '[...] following mechanism may be followed to expedite the development of new drug and approval process'.[33]

Again, the NDCT Rules, 2019, prescribed the process to be followed once the special situation was established. Paragraph 2 (ii) (A) of the Second Schedule explains the Accelerated Approval Process. It states: 'Accelerated approval process may be allowed to a new drug for a disease or condition, taking into account its severity, rarity, or prevalence and the availability or lack of alternative treatments, provided that there is a prima facie case of the product being of meaningful therapeutic benefit over the existing treatment.'[34]

Yet again, these preconditions for considering an accelerated approval for Covid-19 vaccines were in place. The severity, rarity, prevalence and lack of alternatives were the factors to consider here. In fact, the NDCT Rules, 2019, are worded in a way that even one of these four factors would be sufficient for undertaking an accelerated approval process. In the cases of Covishield and Covaxin, not one but all four factors were applicable.

The next regulatory factor was: what stage of the trial should a drug be in to use the authority established under the Second Schedule. Paragraph 2 (ii) (A) (d) established this precondition. It states:

> If the remarkable efficacy is observed with a defined dose in the Phase II clinical trial of investigational new drugs for the unmet medical needs of serious and life threatening diseases in the country, it may be considered for grant of marketing approval by the Central Licencing Authority based on Phase II clinical trial data. In such cases, additional post licensure studies may be required to be conducted after approval to generate the data on larger population to further verify and describe the clinical benefits, as per the protocol approved by the Central Licencing Authority.[35]

This provision makes it clear that emergency authorization could have been taken based on the Phase II clinical trial itself. In the case of Covaxin, partial information was actually available from the Phase III trial at the time of the regulatory approval.

Paragraph Paragraph 2 (ii) (A) (e) describes what data the Central Licensing Authority should look at while considering an approval.

> The type of information needed to demonstrate the potential of a drug to address an unmet medical need will depend on the stage of drug development. Early in development, such potential should be sufficiently demonstrated based on nonclinical models, a mechanistic rationale and pharmacologic data. Later in development, prior to new drug approval such potential should be demonstrated through clinical data to address an unmet medical need.[36]

Yet again, given the stage of the vaccine development, non-clinical models, pharmacological data as well as early clinical trial data was available to the regulators at the time of approving Covaxin.

In the case of Covishield, the popular criticism was whether the bridge trial prescribed by the regulators was sufficient. Stated differently, should the regulator have accounted for the Phase I data from other countries as is? The NDCT Rules, 2019, address this point clearly in the Second Schedule.

Paragraph Paragraph 1 (iv) (b) of the Second Schedule specifies the preconditions that apply to drugs imported from other countries and are not made in India. This paragraph states:

> For new drug substances discovered or developed in countries other than India, Phase I data should be submitted along with the application. After submission of Phase I data generated outside India to the Central Licensing Authority, permission may be granted to repeat Phase I trials or to conduct Phase II trials and subsequently Phase III trials concurrently with other global trials for that drug. For a drug going to be introduced for the first time in the country, Phase III trial may be required to be conducted in India before permission to market the drug is granted unless otherwise exempted.[37]

These guidelines clearly demonstrate that the regulator was well within its rights to accept Phase I trial data from other countries submitted by the SII. The permission of Phase II and Phase III trials could have been granted based on the Phase I data that had been submitted. The guidelines made it possible to undertake Phase II and Phase III trials in India concurrently with other countries.

Finally, the guidelines also state that for a first-time-use in India, the drug *may*—not should—require Phase III trial in India. SII was still asked to conduct local bridging trials. The process was very much in accordance with the guidelines laid down in the Second Schedule of the NDCT Rules, 2019.

As per long-established standard ways of reading guideline documents, the special situations could be applied to all 'eligible' drugs. So it wasn't the case that a vaccine not made in India could not be found suitable for approvals under special situations.

Regulatory Shortfall?

Having established the rigour of the vaccine approval process, there could only have been two potential criticisms to make.

The first potential criticism could be that while the regulator was well within its rights scientifically to do what it did, was the interpretation of the available data correct?

While this could be a theoretical argument, the lacuna in this question is self-evident. Who regulates the regulator? In a democracy, there is an inherent trust established in public institutions. These institutions have a proven track record of dealing with different daunting situations. Even if allegations were to be made that the regulator did not know its job well enough, the burden of proof would be on the individual making the allegation rather than on the regulator to demonstrate its competence.

If this were not the case, what would become of the sanctity of any public institution in the country? The public systems in India work with adequate checks and balances, with different types of institutions taking the lead in different situations based on their primary role and competency. To allege that the political establishment forced a decision on the health regulators without first filtering the argument through the sieve of the NDCT Rules, 2019, could imply ineptitude, vendetta, collusion or malice.

With the benefit of the hindsight of a large, successful public vaccination programme behind us, it can only be hoped that this criticism was born out of either ineptitude or personal vendetta rather than competitor collusion or malice.

The second potential criticism that could have been levelled and should have been more broadly discussed was the following: having satisfied itself with all preconditions and procedural formalities established in the Second Schedule, should the regulator have approved mass vaccination? In other words, could the favourable regulatory outcome following the guidelines of the Second Schedule result in a nationwide vaccine programme, or were the rules intended for a more limited use?

Indeed, one media article did level this criticism.[38] This was perhaps the only opinion piece that went into the details of the NDCT Rules, 2019, while analysing the approval process.

There was some merit in this criticism. The 'Special Situations' guidelines do not mention what kind of use a drug taking the emergency approval route should be subjected to. Sure, the Central Licensing Authority could allow the use of the vaccine, but should it allow the use for the whole country at once? The guidelines do not talk about the countrywide administration of a drug potentially due to the bounded rationality principle—it was not envisaged that the country would have to take up universal adult vaccination for any reason.

2 (ii) (A) (d), which established this precondition, does use the phrase 'may be considered for grant of marketing approval by the Central Licencing Authority'.[39] In this particular case, the approval was for vaccine administration by public authorities rather than marketing by individual firms.

It can also be argued that while the intention of the approval was mass adult vaccination, the actual vaccine administration was still a gradual process. Had there been adverse reactions to the vaccine in a significant number of cases, the programme could well have been rolled back. This option was open to the regulators and to the Ministry of Health and Family Welfare at all times.

Hence, even if there was criticism that the regulator took a discretionary call to allow mass vaccination rather than starting small and gradually and then scaling up slowly, the necessary rollback safeguard was very much available. In reality, the process was very much a gradual ramp-up due to various factors, the most important one being the supply–demand mismatch of the vaccine availability itself. Additionally, public health authorities controlling the process rather than private entities built in an additional layer of trust and dependability.

Ultimately all regulators used this discretion—assessing the known and potential benefits of the vaccine over the known and potential risks. Perhaps the SEC of the CDSCO did not use this exact phrase or an appropriate equivalent text as clearly as it could have in its approval documents and associated media releases.

Eventually, it boiled down to the trust in public institutions. The preponderance of national opinion was to back the vaccination programme. The loud critics who assiduously squat over the mediums of opinion dissemination, however, had pre-determined cavilling arguments ready. Sensational headlines rather than curious, open-minded questioning dominated the cacophony of the public debate. The casualty in this showdown was nuanced criticism and detail-oriented inquiry.

Fortunately for the country, the regulators were right. India's scientists and doctors had done the right thing. It just took an additional effort to get the critics around to overcome their genuine objections and in several cases, conceit. No success matches a mass vaccination success.

7

A STRATEGIC NUMBERS GAME

In the course of routine national immunization programmes, vaccine procurement would typically be a boring exercise. Orders would be negotiated and then money exchanged for the actual vaccine doses. There would be nothing remotely exciting about the process.

Yet, the Covid-19 vaccine ordering approach worldwide was nothing short of a long drama—filled with hope and despair, tragedy and joy, and, in some cases, anger that boiled over to the point of severe harm to bilateral relationships even to the extent of threatening international conflict.

At the bottom of this lay the cold numbers. There are over 8 billion people on the planet. The first vaccination occurred in mid-December 2020, at which point there were already 75 million confirmed Covid-19 cases worldwide—nearly 1 per cent of the entire global population.[1] It is difficult to say how many more were infected and had not been formally tested.

The vaccination count worldwide did not overtake cumulative global cases for another month and a half—at the end of January when the global vaccinations (approximately 110 million) overtook the cumulative global confirmed cases.[2]

At this point, scientists world over were working with the idea of herd immunity. The Mayo Clinic defines the concept of herd immunity as: 'Herd immunity occurs when a large portion of a community (the herd) becomes immune to a disease. The spread of disease from person to person becomes unlikely when herd immunity is achieved. As a result, the whole community becomes protected—not just those who are immune.'[3]

Herd immunity required against a pathogen is directly correlated to its infectiousness. For Covid-19, this was thought to be dependent on the variant, but for even the less virulent B.1.1.7 Alpha variant, it was estimated that only when 80 per cent of the population achieved immunity against the virus would the rest be safe.[4] It was clear, therefore, that during early to mid-2021, the world was far from getting anywhere near herd immunity against Covid-19.

So how did nations respond? Anecdotal evidence show how human relationships and mutual self-interest became the primary drivers.

Heads of State Turn Commercial Negotiators

Israel, a relatively small country by population, was not among the first to place orders. However, then PM Benjamin Netanyahu acted soon after Pfizer/BioNTech announced their Phase III efficacy results in November 2020.[5] Over the course of reportedly 30 phone calls,[6] Netanyahu and Pfizer CEO Albert Bourla made a deal for Israel to acquire vaccines expeditiously, in exchange for a higher price and sharing of vaccine performance data with Pfizer.[7]

Netanyahu was not the only person to negotiate in this manner. Ursula von der Leyen, president of the European Commission and a close friend of the former German Chancellor Angela Merkel, similarly negotiated with Bourla, reportedly over text messages and phone calls in early 2021.[8]

As explained in the earlier parts of this book, ordering vaccines early didn't guarantee deliveries in time. Every sovereign authority was expected to join a queue for a commodity that initially did not exist, then began existing in small quantities for a period of time and finally scaled in production slower than the global requirement.

Even though the EU had placed orders in the middle of 2020, the initial production was slow. Pfizer entirely shut production at its European site in Puurs, Belgium, for two weeks in January 2021 to perform upgrades even when the pandemic ravaged Europe.[9]

Faced days later with production delays of its other major vaccine option, the Oxford/AstraZeneca vaccine,[10] von der Leyen mounted a stringent effort to ensure that the EU would receive vaccines on priority.[11]

Across the Atlantic, newly elected US president Joe Biden did pretty much the same, increasing orders for Pfizer and Moderna vaccines in February[12] and a month later invoking the Cold War era Defense Production Act[13] to ensure a US embargo on exports of either raw material or vaccines until domestic supplies were sufficient.

These actions all had a common theme—the use of leverage and influence with the vaccine producers to negotiate the prioritization of supplies. These actions also underscored the wide gulf in accessibility even where countries ordered vaccines early but lacked the leverage to ensure their early deliveries. It was quite clear that a combination of some levers of power, ability to outspend other countries and using regulatory measures were necessary to access the vaccines, but even this combination was not going to prove sufficient in actual delivery.

When Money Could Not Buy Vaccines

Canada, which placed its first orders for Pfizer/BioNTech vaccines in August 2020, was stuck between a US export embargo and the EU taking similar actions. At one point, it imported Covishield from India,[14] as did the UK. This was a case of supreme irony and antagonistic vaccine nationalism playing out—the US invoking a war-time legislation limiting raw material[15] for Covishield to India was essentially blocking Canadian access to vaccines!

Another example of a rich country facing vaccine access challenges came from across the Pacific. Japan went into the middle of May 2021 with only 1 per cent of its population vaccinated.[16] A deal between the International Olympic Committee, Japan and Pfizer ensured vaccine doses to Olympic participants and organizing staff. This arrangement had to be negotiated despite Japan originally ordering 120 million doses of vaccines in July 2020.[17] At the Opening Ceremony of the Tokyo Olympics, Pfizer's CEO Bourla, who attended as a guest, was hosted at the Akasaka Palace state guest house,[18] typically meant only to host visiting heads of state.

The situation faced by the richest countries—members of the groupings no less than the G-7 and the Organisation for Economic Co-operation and Development—showed clearly that placing early orders did very little.

The earliest recipients leaned on every artefact of leverage they had, from being host to production bases, sources of supplies, to ethnic kinship, paying a premium or controversially trading off their citizens' private medical data to buy vaccines. Nations that could force their case did so by whatever means possible. Those that could not, tried what they could, even implicitly elevating the executive chief of the vaccine manufacturer to a protocol status equivalent to that of a head of state.

Collective Bargaining

For most of the developing world, access to vaccines was historically brokered by major global health initiatives such as the Gavi. These organizations are incredibly important for regular vaccine access to the developing world. In response to Covid-19, the COVAX[19] programme was initiated—a collaboration between Gavi, the CEPI, the WHO and UNICEF.

However, COVAX was not well suited to an urgent mission mode response. It was assembled on the premise that bulk ordering would create a monopsony. Yet again, the failure of such collective bargaining to produce initial early results demonstrated that without non-commercial leverage on pharmaceutical firms, there was precious little by way of influence.[20]

The size of the orders lost all marginal utility, as money was commodified in chasing scarce vaccines. There was always someone else willing to outspend the competition. Also, programmes like COVAX were publicly funded and supported by philanthropic contributions. They depended on production licensing arrangements but did not enable access to vaccine intellectual property.

COVAX could neither facilitate production licensing agreements nor direct purchases at the scale required.[21] The western Covid-19 response was centred on the new mRNA vaccines, which no global vaccine producer had the ability to manufacture at scale without intellectual property and requisite manufacturer support. Importing them would not have been pragmatic, as was discovered in the negotiation process.

In fact, the past experience of Gavi also showed that its success had higher probability when the vaccines were already available or the technology to make the vaccines was well known and it only had to be translated to the final product. An aggregator could bring together short-term funding in the mix by showing a larger order book. But a spike of funding could not accelerate the evolution of technology itself.

This was borne out in a previous situation, too, where Gavi had tried to change the trivalent polio vaccine regime (three oral doses as is the common practice) to a bivalent one (two oral doses), followed by an injectable polio vaccine. However, despite the disease being well known, the injectable polio vaccine had to be developed from scratch. This could not be done, and Gavi was unable to help bring this switch in the administration of polio vaccines.[22]

It is no surprise that a well-intentioned and reasonably well-funded programme did not work in the case of Covid-19. If India had relied on such third-party networks, it would have taken too long to deliver a very limited supply of vaccines to more than a billion people. They would have also competed against other less fortunate citizens of the developing world.

India did not rely on this option for its vaccine procurement.

The India Way

It is in this context that India's approach to vaccine procurement should be evaluated. The popular conception peddled for months that India did not throw money at the vaccines was not just ill-informed, it also lacked the understanding of how vaccines falling under the category of medical goods were manufactured and their production ramped up.

India responded in a manner that was a clean break from the past, focussing on the nation's strengths, while also in the process replicating the human factor and decisive top-down action. Response to a crisis is a function of the available options, and India had very few options available. A retrospective view of the actions taken demonstrate a very interesting aatmanirbhar approach, focussed on maximizing domestic potential to successfully deal with the crisis.

If India had to administer up to 3 billion vaccine doses as quickly as the West, it was clear that the only choice was to leverage domestic vaccine development and production capability. India had to make sure that Indian firms got everything that was needed to develop and produce vaccines quickly.

That is exactly what India did.

The government response focussed on playing to our strengths, while focussing on eliminating every hurdle in the way of accelerated development. Every interested producer was encouraged to take their path of choice, with a proactive assertion that the government would give them whatever support they needed.

What the central government identified very early on was the importance of placing a proactive supporting role provided by one central decision-making authority. Aided by PM Modi's empowered task force, the focus was on quick decision-making to first get the vaccines ready and approved for use following all guidelines. In contrast, the delays were partly attributed to each country needing to sign off on an order.[23]

India's Process Facilitation

India's focus remained on process facilitation. Once the vaccines got approved in India, the government could keep placing orders with the manufacturers to fulfil their expansion plans with reasonable forward visibility. The government would not have to commit billions of dollars in advance, while the manufacturers got full process support from the former in lieu of the initial risk capital they were putting in towards research and development.

Indian drug and vaccine manufacturers proved competent at creating sturdy products at reasonable costs. Bharat Biotech spent ₹530 crore (approximately $70 million) on the development of Covaxin.[24] Zydus Cadila spent ₹400–500 crore (approximately $53–$66 million).[25] Despite different technologies, the costs were not orders of magnitude apart.

Part of this funding came from the ₹900 crore granted by the Government of India under Mission Covid Suraksha[26] announced on 29 November 2020. This programme implemented outlays for three separate categories through requests for expressions of interest (REOI):

REOI-1: Development of Covid-19 vaccine candidates
REOI-2: Enhancement of capacity to support Covid-19 vaccine development
REOI-3: Enhancing capacity for conduct of human clinical trials for Covid-19 vaccine candidates.[27]

The DBT received a total of 66 proposals across these three categories with ₹710 crore (approximately $94 million) committed by early 2021.[28] Notable in Mission Covid Suraksha was the focus on investing in logistics and organizational details ahead of time.

An interesting Right to Information (RTI) request sought to understand where exactly each rupee of this corpus went. In particular, some press sources insisted that since ₹900 crore were not fully spent, Mission Covid Suraksha was a failure.[29]

Success or failure is established from the overall result, not the completion of a small intermediate step. As of mid-July 2022, India hit 2 billion vaccinations. The US, Canada and all of Europe, which together host the vast multinational western Big Pharma production base for Covid-19 vaccines, performed 1.95 billion cumulative vaccinations at exactly the same time.[30]

In other words, India's efforts over time ensured single-handed production of exactly the same quantity of vaccines as the total produced by large blocs. And it must be remembered that India began large-scale vaccinations on 1 March 2021, three months after these countries. In the 15 months since, India had caught up with their entire combined production volume to date, despite being bogged down by a natural resource crunch relative to the western world.

By stepping in and establishing the framework through which all companies with vaccine candidates could execute their multiphase trials, the government essentially eliminated this responsibility from the hands of the companies themselves. While all major nations leveraged their publicly funded medical research and coordination establishment to support vaccine development, the Indian approach was unique in the manner in which the DBT and CSIR exercised pervasive and highly effective control over the trials process.[31]

The result was that the Indian vaccine trials and ordering process were unique in several ways. It is indisputable that the costs of development and trailing were orders of magnitude cheaper than any other benchmark in the West and in a much shorter time frame.

India's Procurement Costs and Process

A natural question that all stakeholders wanted answered was the total cost of procurement of vaccines by India. All the information was made publicly available and was reported in the mainstream media. In fact, the authors had been collecting this information over the course of a year prior to this book being written.

The order dates and the quantities for the two main vaccine suppliers, SII and Bharat Biotech, are shown below:

TABLE 6

Procurement from Serum Institute of India and Bharat Biotech[32]

Serum Institute of India			
Date	*Order Size (in crore)*	*Price/Dose**	*Order Cost*
11 Jan 2021	1.1	₹210	₹231 crore
3 February 2021	1	₹210	₹210 crore
17 March 2021	10	₹157.50	₹1,575 crore
28 April 2021	11	₹157.50	₹1,732.50 crore
8 June 2021	25	₹157.50	₹3,937.50 crore
16 July 2021	37.5	₹215.25	₹8,071.88 crore
9 September 2021	66	₹215.25	₹14,206.50 crore

Bharat Biotech			
Date	*Order Size (in crore)*	*Price/Dose**	*Order Cost*
11 January 2021	0.55	₹295.00	₹115.00 crore
19 January 2021	0.45	₹300.00	₹135.00 crore
17 March 2021	2	₹300.00	₹600.00 crore
28 April 2021	5	₹157.50	₹787.50 crore
8 June 2021	19	₹157.50	₹2,992.50 crore
16 July 2021	28.5	₹225.75	₹6,433.88 crore

*Dose cost includes 5 per cent Goods and Services Tax (GST)

Thus, the total all-inclusive order cost involving Covishield was just under ₹30,000 crore for over 150 crore doses. Similarly, total orders for Covaxin were just over ₹11,000 crore for 55.5 crore doses.[33]

In addition, the central government made two orders for Corbevax of 30 crore and 5 crore doses. The first was an advance payment of ₹1,500 crore[34] to aid rapid development and productization, while the latter was a conventional order priced at ₹152.25 per dose (inclusive of GST) for a total order size of ₹761.25 crore[35].

Finally, Zydus Cadila received an order for 1 crore doses and needle-free applicators valued at ₹375.90 crore (inclusive of GST).[36]

Several observations can be made from these numbers. The topline picture is that a total of over 240 crore (2.43 billion) doses had been ordered till June 2022. Their aggregate cost was under ₹45,000 crore ($5.75 billion). Up to 17 July 2022, 200 crore (2 billion) vaccinations were carried out, and approximately 14 crore doses remained part of the pending supply, i.e. domestic production already supplied till September-end was approximately 203 crore (2.03 billion) doses out of the 240 crore total doses ordered.[37]

A further analysis of the order sequence shows a very interesting trend: during 2021, when the controversy about 'lack of orders' peaked, the government was placing orders approximately every six to eight weeks. It was progressively ordering larger volumes, very closely aligned to actual production levels.

For example, the SII produced over 100 million doses of Covishield in June 2021.[38] At the start of the same month, the SII received a fresh order of just over twice the dynamic production rate.

This trend was visible repeatedly in the ordering process through 2021—until the situation was well under control, the government deliberately chose to place orders equivalent to approximately a two-month supply of the dynamic production rate at the time. This continued until the autumn of 2021, when large orders for Covishield and Covaxin corresponding to multiple months of production volume were placed.

An obvious question that arises is, 'Why were orders placed in this manner? Why didn't the Indian government front-load very large orders to ensure production?'

The reason is easy if one considers how the government tried to solve the multivariate equation involving the ability of the vaccine makers to scale and deliver, the possibility of new vaccines coming up and the financial outlay made in the Union Budget for the financial year 2021–22.

While Covishield and Covaxin were approved at the very beginning of the year, there was still a significant possibility that Corbevax from Biological E and ZyCov-D from Zydus Cadila would clear their clinical trials expeditiously. What would the government do if they placed extremely high-value orders for Covishield and Covaxin early in 2021, but then other vaccines cleared trials sooner than expected? They would have vaccines that they could not find funds to place immediate orders for. The government had ₹35,000 crore allocated in the Union Budget in February 2021, plus smaller amounts from other sources, including the Prime Minister's Citizen Assistance and Relief in Emergency Situations (PM-CARES) fund.

The government strove extremely hard to keep aggregate order costs to a figure that adds up to the total funding it had set aside or obtained in 2021—and succeeded. However, throughout the process of placing orders during the early months of 2021, it was always compelled to make sure that it never ordered any vaccine in such a large order size that it was left with too little to immediately allocate to any new vaccine producer with an urgent capital infusion requirement.

Further, it was able to fund a significant part of its Covid-19 vaccine production capabilities from internal resources, along with funds from the Indian government and Gavi. Through the whole of 2021, SII continued to scale up vaccine production more or less at the rate at which it estimated it would manage.

Similarly, Bharat Biotech received ₹65 crore in funding to scale up its production facilities in Hyderabad and Bengaluru, in addition to accessing not just one but three vaccine production public sector undertakings (PSUs): Haffkine Biopharmaceutical Corporation Ltd, Indian Immunologicals Ltd and Bharat Immunologicals and Biologicals Ltd.[39] Each of these PSUs received central grants to augment and set aside production capability to produce Covaxin.

This was done because Covaxin had particular scaling constraints quite unlike Covishield—it needed BSL-3 facilities to cultivate the live Covid-19 virus before it was killed and used to produce the vaccine. Not only did this add a production bottleneck but it also posed the risk of a lab leak that could be the devastating source of an outbreak. In addition, the government brokered an agreement between Bharat Biotech and Panacea Biotec, since these were the only private sector companies with BSL-3 facilities at the time.

By leveraging and brokering a collaboration amongst a number of public and private sector entities that had the physical infrastructure required to produce Covaxin, the Indian government facilitated the production of this vaccine in a far more effective manner than what it would have managed by simply writing out a large cheque to Bharat Biotech in early 2021 and then leaving the company to figure out the rest on its own.

The government supported Biological E with an advance purchase order, facilitating its trials and production. Additionally, active support from the DBT-BIRAC enabled Zydus Cadila to achieve EUA for Zycov-D in August 2021[40]—the first DNA-based vaccine for Covid-19 in the world. Soon afterwards, Zycov-D received its first order at the end of October 2021.

With all these facts viewed retrospectively, the government's ordering game plan became much clearer: it worked with a careful eye on the total fund corpus it had. It knew that some producers had more upfront support requirements than others. It was careful not to overcommit to long-term orders of Covishield and Covaxin, not because it didn't believe in them but because it had a continuous line of communication with the companies, making it clear that successive orders would be placed on a predictable schedule tied to their production rate—which is what happened. This gave them the ability to make large advance funding commitments where required—whether it was an advance order to Biological E, or funding to various PSUs to augment their BSL-3 facilities in order to produce Covaxin. By carefully tailoring its approach to the specific technical requirements of each vaccine maker, it was able to therefore maximize the return on its investment. By the end of the year 2021, India had four authorized vaccines and, more critically, each and every one of them had a local production line.

Money vs Results: Real World Outcomes

For the US as well as the EU, the order quantities eventually reached several times the size of their total population. Other high-income countries did the same—with the UK and Canada each placing orders totalling five to six times their population.[41] At the first glance, this seems like exactly what was needed—decisive action by the governments backed by effectively a blank cheque to innovate.

Based on this assumption, the Indian government was roundly criticized for putting in piecemeal orders. On the one hand, the measured Indian approach was criticized for being nothing close to a blank cheque. On the other hand, there was also a criticism in 2021 that vaccine makers should not profiteer from a crisis, often by the same critics.

The governments in North America and Europe were largely spared of such polemical criticism, despite the fact that their blank cheques did not result in the expected vaccine delivery outcomes.

It is instructive to look at the data here: how many vaccines were ordered and delivered as of early 2022? For simplicity, we will compare three entities—North America (the US, Canada and Mexico), Europe (the EU, all non-EU/ European Economic Area countries plus the British Isles) and India.

TABLE 7

Vaccine Orders and Administration[42]

Entity	*Order Total*	*Administered (till July 2022)*
North America	2,350 million	1.03 billion
Europe	4,600 million	1.30 billion
India	2,390 million	2 billion

The data is clear—till mid-2022, India administered more vaccines than either North America or Europe, using about 1.6 billion doses of Covishield and 340 million doses of Covaxin.[43] With approximately the same number of total orders as North America, India administered almost twice as many doses. The data shows that the approach of ordering massive quantities of vaccines ahead of time did not guarantee their administration.

The enormous spending did not generate a commensurately large production volume either. At the most, the high initial financial commitments enabled the West to start approximately a month earlier and generated early volumes higher than the Indian production rate in the first quarter of 2021. But this did not last. By the second quarter of 2021 (April–June), India had overtaken combined North American output and was catching up to Europe. By the third and fourth quarters of 2021, India was producing well over half a billion vaccines per quarter, exceeding Europe and North America combined. This trend continued in the first quarter of 2022.

Quarterly Vaccinations: India vs Continents*

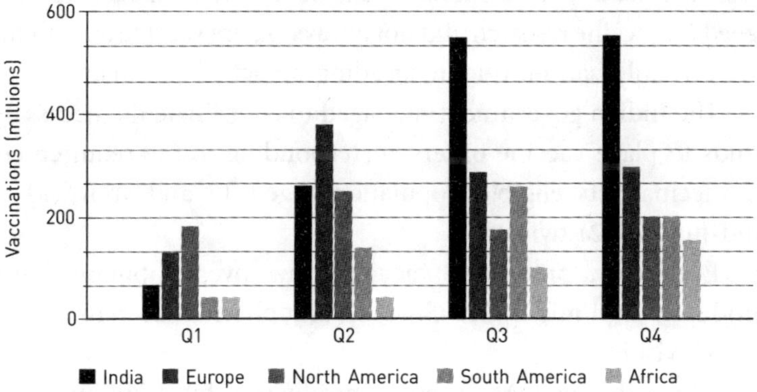

**Source:* 'Our World in Data', https://bit.ly/3DRRRGI. Accessed on 11 November 2022.

In hindsight, simply by writing blank cheques, the governments in the West did not drive significantly different outcomes. Viewed strictly as a return on investment exercise, western spending on vaccine development was incredibly costly and wasteful. Throwing vast amounts of money at the problem enabled parallelization of vaccine trials. But eventually it did not yield more vaccine candidates, did not impact speed of delivery, except perhaps for one quarter, and eventually did not enable greater production volume.

Time Is the Best Judge

In January 2021, as vaccinations started being administered across the world, India was one of the select geographies alongside China, the US, the UK and the EU, which had more than one vaccine option to rely on. Russia only had a single option in Sputnik V. However, both the developed West and India would encounter a common problem approximately two months into general vaccination—demand outstripping early supply and production scaling. Looking back at the various global experiences, it became clear that making more money available to vaccine makers did not speed up vaccine research, did not always ensure vaccine availability and certainly had no role in speeding up actual vaccination.

The Indian government managed to coordinate the necessary funds to place vaccine orders corresponding to the requirement to vaccinate its eligible population (aged 12 and above as of mid-June 2022) twice.

Eventually, only four vaccines saw over a billion doses produced until mid-2022—Sinovac, Sinopharm, Pfizer/BioNTech and Covishield.

When the total AstraZeneca production hit 2 billion doses, Covishield alone accounted for 1.7 billion doses. The SII crossed the 1-billion mark for Covishield by November 2021.[44] The India-made Covishield formulation far exceeded the parent producer in volume, by nearly four to one. AstraZeneca had stated that its manufacturing spawned across 25 sites in 15 countries.[45]

The total production of Covaxin as of mid-June 2022 was around 35 crore (350 million) doses, counting domestic production and exports. The total production of the Moderna mRNA vaccine in the US as of mid-June 2022 was just under 300 million vaccine doses.[46] In other words, Covaxin had already exceeded the American production rate of the Moderna vaccine, which was supported by far greater financial resources. Additionally, the available data also suggests that Covaxin production in India exceeded the combined EU and UK production of AstraZeneca.

The front loading of vaccine orders, in fact, may have had a demonstrable negative impact. The aggressive early spending left money in the hands of vaccine producers who did not always deliver. But more critically, that money was no longer accessible for urgent current and future requirements of the government. For example, in March 2022, the US was curtailing booster vaccine doses because it did not have enough funding to pay for everyone's doses.[47]

While it is true that the West has offered booster doses to a much larger share of its population than India, it is also true that India exceeds both North America and Europe in terms of the population that has been administered at least one dose—and the Indian share keeps rising faster. This means the West has one section of population that is vaccinated thrice, but a larger share than India that is not vaccinated *at all*, and due to social, religious or political reasons, refuses to be vaccinated. Correspondingly, the US and other western countries have seen regular Covid-19 outbreaks because these populations intermingle in public.

In comparison, Indian urban areas were almost saturated in terms of vaccination cover by mid-2022. The areas with lower vaccination coverage in India are characterized not by political beliefs as in the West, but by geographical remoteness. The same remoteness also protects the residents from contact. As a result, since early 2022, when India rapidly achieved high levels of vaccination coverage, it has sustained a relatively low active caseload and few localized and contained outbreaks.

8

GETTING THE PLUMBING RIGHT

'*Akramenānupāyena karmārambho na sidhyati*'[1] is a Sanskrit phrase from a text that coaches the readers on personal conduct in life. It means: 'A work begun with no order and means does not succeed.'

A national vaccination plan without the understanding of how to start and end was going to be a non-starter. The Covid-19 pandemic also presented several unique problems to address.

A Multifaceted Problem

The first and most obvious challenge was scale. Scale is a defining feature of how India works. Indian public policy is unique in that it has to manage the unparalleled scale of Indian population and geography. There are no templates and no best practices, which may fit as solutions to the problems born out of the sheer size and enormity of numbers in India.

In an alarmist 1968 book, American biologist and Malthusian Paul R. Ehrlich had rather derogatorily described India after his 1966 visit as a country full of people. 'The streets seemed alive with people. People eating, people washing, people sleeping. People visiting, arguing, and screaming. People thrusting their hands through the taxi window, begging. People defecating and urinating. People clinging to buses. People herding animals. People, people, people, people.'[2]

While Ehrlich's doomsday predictions about India on account

of its population and the lack of social infrastructure were long proved incorrect, his characterization captured the present-day dilemma for vaccination planning. Alhough the state capacity had significantly improved since the time he visited India in the decade of food shortages and military conflicts, clearly reaching out potentially to 1.37 billion people for vaccination was not going to be easy.

The second challenge came from the global nature of the Covid-19 pandemic. It was clear that to enable people to travel, some kind of a proof of vaccination would be needed. While it was unclear what approaches different countries would adopt, what was clear from the outset was that every administration had to be adequately recorded and made easily retrievable. Such a 'record, retrieve and validate' requirement was going to be integral for movement of Indians within and outside the country.

The vaccination process would have to be such that all state governments within the country felt comfortable with the guarantee of some type of a central standardization. When people crossed borders within the country by road, rail, air or water, the movement had to be easy, predictable and costless from the perspective of public health.

When Indians travelled abroad, the destination countries would have to feel comfortable with the Indian vaccination programme and its delivery apart from their effectiveness. This was a key consideration at the time vaccines were being developed, as there were multiple voices in each country on how the international movement should be handled. While no government really knew what the right answer was, there were enough indications that such movement was not going to be barrier-free. The term 'vaccine passport' was finding increasing use in international public lexicon, though the idea dated back to the plague year of 1897.[3]

The third challenge was the readiness to take vaccines. While the example of pulse polio and, more recently, the infant immunization programmes showed that the vaccine delivery process can run at a certain scale, the Covid-19 situation was unprecedented. This was not about covering all Indians, it involved covering every adult.

This posed a key challenge—consent. An infant getting the prescribed vaccine doses within Mission Indradhanush—India's immunization programme for children up to five years of age, which also includes an oral dose of the polio vaccine—essentially had no choice. They were enrolled in the vaccination programme by default and could not say no. But the adults could say no and, in fact, the null hypothesis had to be that many, if not most adults, would say no.

There were many reasons for this null hypothesis. There was no real precedent of any mass adult vaccination programme in India. The statistics from the vaccination effort against the 1897 plague were not well known. More recently, during the swine flu outbreak in 2009, the same players—SII, Bharat Biotech, Zydus Cadila and Panacea Biotec—had worked on various vaccine efforts. But these did not see a lot of acceptance.[4]

At that time, the state of Maharashtra had been the worst affected by the outbreak of swine flu. The state had offered free vaccine doses to certain segments of the population, such as pregnant women. But only 2 per cent of the intended segment took the vaccine, without a proper understanding of the need, benefits, risks and a general awareness about the concept of vaccinations for adults.[5]

It was going to be an uphill battle combating vaccine hesitancy born out of ignorance, complacency, mistrust or personal beliefs.

The fourth issue was a derivative problem of various other hurdles. Developing vaccine acceptance within society was going to be fundamental to reducing the burden of the highly communicable disease. If a significant number of Indians did not opt for the vaccine, it would reduce the social benefit of the vaccination programme in its entirety.

No one was safe until everyone was safe. But if a significant proportion of society chose not to accept the safety of the Covid-19 vaccines, it would mean higher exposure and higher risk to these individuals, which could result in the potentially reduced impact of vaccines on those vaccinated. This scenario was possible because the virus could mutate in the bodies of unvaccinated individuals, with new mutations potentially escaping the vaccine protection cover.

This externality could have a detrimental impact on India's fight against Covid-19 and could well render the whole effort meaningless. It would be very difficult for society itself to internalize this externality and solve the issue via mutual bargaining. This situation was akin to the negative production costs in economics—the marginal social cost of failure would be significantly higher than the marginal private cost.

The situation would need active government participation and management and could not be left to the 'market'—in this case every Indian citizen—to correct itself through a consultative process and through the power of influence.

The fifth problem was that of time. It was important to complete the vaccination process in the shortest possible time to ensure economic and social normalcy in the coming years. While the government understood that the financial year 2020–21, which ran from 1 April 2020 till 31 March 2021, was going to see a sharp decline in economic activity, the economic stagnation could not be allowed to be carried over to the next financial year.

The strict lockdown of March 2020, which extended with progressively reducing severity till June 2020 and was then necessary to prepare the medical infrastructure, took its economic toll. The gross domestic product (GDP) in the first quarter of financial year 2020–21 sharply declined by 23.9 per cent in the estimate that came out on 31 August 2020.[6]

Although this reading was revised upward in later estimates, it was amply clear that lockdowns could not be a solution to combat the virus. The vaccines had to be administered quickly to keep any future economic damage manageable.

The sixth consideration was that of medical personnel. There had to be enough trained medical personnel available when the vaccination programme rolled out to ensure coverage of the entire population.

India's medical infrastructure has a three-tier architecture. Healthcare is a subject in the State List. These subjects are defined and enlisted under List II of the Seventh Schedule of the Constitution of India.[7] Hence, they are the exclusive domain of each state government. This list effectively also excludes the central government from framing any new laws under these subjects.

The central government, hence, had to use the power of persuasion to prepare the medical infrastructure across states for effective vaccination delivery. It had to ensure that the individual capacities of the state governments, which unsurprisingly varied widely, should not become an impediment in the success of the vaccination programme.

The seventh and not the least problematic issue was that of finances. The government had to decide how the financial model for vaccine administration would work. The optimal sharing of the financial burden between the central government, the state governments and the private individuals had to be arrived at.

While the market costs of vaccines weren't clear until the fourth quarter of 2020, there were some initial suggestions in the industry that the mRNA vaccines may cost between $20 and $30 per dose.[8] On the other hand, the SII had talked about a pricing of $3 per dose for their vaccine. What was not clear in the third quarter of 2020 was the choice of vaccine—the government had to prepare for all eventualities in the planning phase.

If a two-dose mRNA vaccine was to be chosen, it would cost $50 just for the vaccine procurement per person. For a billion Indians, this would mean a cost of $50 billion (approximately ₹375,000 crore). This was the upper extreme of potential costs.

If the SII's Covishield became available at the stated price, the government would have had to shell out $6 per person or $6 billion (approximately ₹45,000 crore) to pick up the tab all by itself.

The cost of actual administration was on top of the vaccine procurement costs. But the budgetary range for the vaccine procurement itself was a hefty $6–$50 billion. This was not a small number from the perspective of annual budgeting, which was already reeling under an economic shock.

The Four Ps behind Vaccination

All these significant and cross-functional challenges required interventions on four counts—process, people, platform and persuasion.

The National Expert Group on Vaccination (NEGVAC) was tasked not just to monitor the development of vaccines themselves, it also took up foundational activities, creating the right plumbing essential to keep the flow of the vaccination process smooth.

The NEGVAC was co-chaired[9] by Dr V.K. Paul of NITI Aayog and secretary, Ministry of Health and Family Welfare. The members of this group included state government representatives from the largest state in each region—Uttar Pradesh from the north, Maharashtra from the west, Tamil Nadu from the south, Assam from the east and Madhya Pradesh from central India. The government experts included representatives from the AIIMS, National Technical Advisory Group on Immunization, secretaries from the Ministry of External Affairs, Department of Expenditure, Department of Biotechnology and the Ministry of Electronics and Information Technology.[10] The group also tapped into a large number of sector and domain specialists.

Essentially, the NEGVAC acted like a body for practical churning on all issues that were likely to come up in India's vaccination journey.[11] This group was constituted on 8 August 2020 and first met on 12 August 2020, when the vaccines were still going through stages of trials.[12] The four Ps had to be addressed a priori and in a well-coordinated manner.

These four aspects were completely interconnected. Without the use of the right technology platform and proper tracking of individual vaccinations, it would not be impossible to run a smooth process. The process also had to build trust, so that individuals didn't shy away from vaccines and, in fact, embraced the relatively unknown medication. One of the key aspects of the process was to have trained and qualified medical personnel fronting every vaccination location.

From Known Knowns to Unknown Unknowns

India is united by national iconography and a sense of purpose. But how would these abstract ideas translate to a national healthcare programme? How would the government build trust during a pandemic while actively battling the sceptics? To complicate the situation further, the scepticism itself would not be uniform in its origin—there would be scepticism of callousness and ignorance or based on fear, beliefs and inducements

In this environment, it was not practical or possible to create an ideal model of a national vaccination process. The process had to factor in all exceptions, and there would, undoubtedly, be several exceptions in such a mass adult vaccination programme. The design had to be flexible enough to accommodate manageable differences of opinions and nudge the sceptics.

It was quite clear from the outset that the vaccines would be approved in emergency use mode only. This meant that the vaccine would not be prescribed by doctors, but would only be administered in specific settings.

The government's decisions had to address the classic trilemma of uncertainty. There were 'known knowns'—issues like skilling and training, requirement of cold chain for vaccine transportation, the population numbers by state, district and village. Then, there were the 'known unknowns'—the dates for vaccine availability, requirement for disposable syringes and vaccine hesitancy issues. Finally, there were the 'unknown unknowns'—which vaccines would India actually get to use, would there be another wave of Covid-19 and if so, when?

Readiness had to be assessed keeping in mind all three types of variables, often leading to either contradictory requirements or layers of redundancies to deal with different situations on the ground.

What would Day 1 look like—the day after the vaccines got authorized for use? This question had to be answered well before Day 1 arrived. It was when the vaccination process hit the road and yet remained flexible enough to make adjustments to the ground realities. This was a perfect example of how bounded rationality was a natural limitation to policymaking. And yet, the policymaking had to cross a minimum threshold of rationality to account for the most plausible situations. Day 1 had to be envisaged by the NEGVAC almost immediately.

Since vaccines were going to be in short supply, their use had to be prioritized. The key objectives of the vaccination programme had to be reduction of morbidity and mortality. The vaccination programme also had to be an enabler of society returning to normalcy. This meant that services that were essential and could not be run without human intervention had to be kept functional or rejuvenated through effective vaccination.

These considerations were the same as recommended by the Values Framework of the Strategic Advisory Group of Experts on Immunization (SAGE) of the WHO. In a report published on 13 November 2020, this body made recommendations on what the priority group selection should be, based on a number of factors.[13]

During a pandemic, the member countries followed the WHO guidelines—a key role of the organization was to guide the world through health crises. The SAGE recommendations were, however, more of an exercise in scenario analysis rather than clear guidance. The guidelines were too broad to be contextually useful and too abstract to be immediately implemented.

However, the lesson most countries took from these guidelines was to focus on vulnerable sections of the society. From the US to the UK to the EU to India, every administration translated the SAGE recommendations to their own setting.

The most important aspect was to start communicating with the states and preparing them for the mass vaccination. Ultimately, India's healthcare delivery remained in the hands of the states. This is where the preparatory work started.

States already had databases on individuals with comorbidities, which were created through non-communicable disease screenings done by health and wellness centres.[14] Many states had these databases digitized. The states were also asked to identify frontline healthcare workers, people with comorbidities and those above 60 years of age. Although the sequencing of who gets the vaccine first was finally determined in January 2021, the initial thought process centred on the standard view that was evolving around the world.

The central government asked the states to start training vaccinators and cold chain handlers. All the people related to vaccine administration, including operational staff, were to be trained following a standard protocol. The government also planned on maintaining a technology system—Immunization Training Management System—that would record the details of all trained individuals for the vaccination programme.[15]

Cold Chain: An Important Consideration

It was important to train the cold chain handlers because it was not clear what temperature would need to be maintained at the end point. While there was a clear understanding that the cold chain would have to be maintained till end point, the actual needs would vary depending on the type of vaccine in use. Hence, states were also asked to identify locations for vaccination where it would be possible to maintain the cold chain. In many states, the cold chain equipment had to be repaired and the states were asked to ensure such efforts were taken up on priority.[16]

While the vaccines India deployed ended up being stored and used at room-grade refrigeration, this was not obvious at all at the time of planning. The cold chain planning turned out to be a classic example of how an issue that takes a lot of mindspace in the preparatory phase of a large programme does not end up being the main constraint. The work done on understanding, refining and preparing a nationwide cold chain for the vaccines was nothing short of exemplary and will doubtless be useful for the country if another need arises to inoculate the nation. This is an instructive story simply because the planning worked very well and nothing went wrong. In public policy decisions, it is often easier to criticize what does not work than it is to praise what works. Human minds are tuned to identify exceptions—a deviation from the mean. Identifying discrepancies does not require specialized knowledge in any field. A simple observation of data is sufficient to observe anomalies. But when complex processes work exactly as planned, there isn't much analysis of why things worked the way they were supposed to. Such observation would require detailed understanding of a process and the components of its corresponding activities.

Cold chains worked in India for Covid-19 vaccination as a result of the investment in this field made through the Electronic Vaccine Intelligence Network or eVIN. Introduced in 2015, this investment predated Covid-19 by several years, and the strength of this network was duly leveraged for the Covid-19 vaccination process.

This was the first area of focus because the vaccines had to be carried in a usable and storage-friendly form. In a single vaccination drive on 31 January 2021, India administered more than 100 million polio vaccinations.[17] From the experience of the mass polio vaccination programmes, the cold chain necessity had been well established. The Covid-19 vaccines also required different types of cold chains based on the type of vaccines.[18]

Protein subunit vaccines such as Novavax, which was being planned to be sold as Covavax in India, vector vaccines such as Covishield that used adenoviruses, inactivated virus vaccines such as Covaxin and DNA-based vaccine planned by Zydus Cadila required temperatures between 2°C and 8°C for transportation and storage. RNA-based vaccines, like the ones from Pfizer and Moderna, required -70°C cold chains. Although the RNA-based vaccines were not likely to form the basis of India's vaccination programme, efforts were still made to provide for the possibility of using them.

Mission Indradhanush was launched on 25 December 2014 as a good governance initiative by then Minister of Health and Family Welfare, J.P. Nadda, who had been working on expanding the immunization coverage. The programme aimed to cover the breadth of immunization, covering all children across India, as well as the depth of immunization, bringing new mandatory vaccines in the national vaccination portfolio.

This programme evolved significantly over the years. The proof that the programme was working was already seen in the declining infant as well as maternal mortality rates.[19]

One of the objectives of the UIP, Comprehensive Multi-Year Plan 2018–2022,[20] was to 'establish a reliable cold chain system to the health facility level'.This programme document stated the rapid progress made by India on managing vaccine cold chains.

The vast scale of India's UIP is supported by more than 27,000 functional cold chain points, of which 750 (3 per cent) are located at district level and above. The remaining 95 per cent are located below the district level, including 76,000 cold chain equipment, 2.5 million health workers and 55,000 cold chain staff. The document further added that approximately 390 million doses are administered annually at 9 million sessions held across the country to immunize 26 million children and 30 million pregnant women.[21]

Vaccine cold chains ensure higher safety, greater availability and retain the potency of the vaccines. These factors together build trust in the efficacy of the vaccine. The National Cold Chain and Vaccine Management Resource Centre in New Delhi and the National Cold Chain Resource Centre in Pune were established in 2013 by the central government in partnership with UNICEF and Government of Maharashtra. With the launch of Mission Indradhanush, these centres got involved in creating this district- and centre-level health infrastructure, which involved physical infrastructure as well as human capital training and capacity building.

The eVIN was strengthened as an outcome of the mid-year review of the previous Comprehensive Multi-Year Plan 2013–2017. This review, undertaken in 2015, focussed on using technology to improve the vaccination process. Enhanced surveillance tools, such as Adverse Event Following Immunization (AEFI), and information on Vaccine Preventable Diseases were developed on the eVIN.

This electronic network was piloted in 12 states in 2015—Assam, Bihar, Chhattisgarh, Gujarat, Himachal Pradesh, Jharkhand, Madhya Pradesh, Manipur, Nagaland, Odisha, Rajasthan and Uttar Pradesh. Since then, the National Health Mission has focussed on expanding the usage of this platform across the country.

It connected four levels of vaccine tracking and availability information on a technology platform—vaccine cold chain end point, district- and regional-level, state-level and national-level centres and stores. The technology platform gave visibility to the healthcare workers on vaccine availability and tracking during transportation. It helped in better understanding the problems of cold chain end points or storage centres. The eVIN introduced the tracking of real-time temperature information of the cold chain equipment across all the vaccine storage cold chain points. It enabled the digitization of the cold chain temperatures, vaccine stocks and flows, and ensured real-time data availability at nearly 10,500 vaccine stores and cold chain points in all 371 districts of the 12 states. Nearly 700 training programmes were implemented for more than 17,000 cold chain handlers and vaccine store managers. Over 2 million transactions were made on the platform every month capturing essential information such as vaccine issues, receipts, discards and transfers. More than 14,000 data loggers were installed for real-time remote temperature monitoring of the cold chain equipment.

The cold chain planning was built on this existing infrastructure. The government mapped out the tehsil-level cold chain situation and encouraged states to fill in the gaps where they existed. The Covid-19 vaccination programme would be significantly larger than India's usual annual vaccination activity. Hence, the need for additional transportation and storage was established and communicated to the states.[22]

India's Federal Spirit

The states, on their part, were also preparing for the programme. While the approach to dividing the responsibilities between the central and the state governments was still evolving, the latter had to do their share of heavy lifting as well, given that they controlled and operated most of the health infrastructure.

Chhattisgarh[23] was one of the pilot states for the eVIN. The state mapped out its requirement of end points for the cold chain and identified that it needed to set up 80 such facilities in addition to the 530 operational cold chain points.

Ladakh,[24] India's newest union territory formed just over a year before the pandemic, prepared by recognizing the unique challenges it was likely to face. Tough terrain, remote villages and limited human capital meant that all arms of the administration—

police, financial planning, healthcare, transport, education and information—had to come together to work with singular zeal towards the national objective. The administration created deeply decentralized committees and task forces to plan the vaccination process at the level of small agglomerations of population, which was very common in Ladakh.

Goa,[25] a small state with thinly spread population but tough physical terrain, planned very early on for availability of syringes in addition to compiling the district-wise population lists. Such practical thinking on part of the state governments would come in very handy during the vaccination programme.

Karnataka[26] identified the actual vaccination sites very early on. It relied on the CHCs and PHCs, and identified more than 29,000 vaccine sites that could work with an unbroken cold chain. The state also identified more than 10,000 vaccinators and ensured that their upcoming responsibilities were properly communicated and the requisite training given.

In Maharashtra, the Mumbai airport[27] authorities planned extensively for the movement of the vaccines. Mumbai airport was to be an important hub for vaccine movement. It is not just well connected with the rest of the country, but its proximity to Pune meant that SII's vaccine production intended for international markets would travel through the Mumbai airport. The airport also had Asia's biggest import cold chain capacity, with a storage capacity of more than 30,000 tonnes. The airport introduced cooltainers to transport vaccines from cold storage areas to the aircraft at the designated temperature. The airport also planned for dedicated docking stations for trucks and X-ray machines to clear the vaccine-related cargo on priority.

Odisha[28] worked on preparing comprehensive lists of frontline and healthcare workers, who were likely to be the first beneficiaries of the vaccine rollout. Different government departments were mobilized to get details of doctors, nurses, other medical workers, Anganwadi workers, social workers, helpers and sanitation workers. This process also effectively signalled to these professionals that they should be ready to take the vaccine.

In Tamil Nadu,[29] the director of Public Health and Preventive Medicine worked with the health officials to prepare a micro plan, covering district-level health centres, PHCs as well as the health sub-centres. The state prepared by understanding the target population to be covered at different levels of the health infrastructure. The officials worked on preparing age distribution-wise potential vaccine beneficiaries at different levels to plan better for the logistics required.

On 20 November 2020, PM Modi reviewed the preparation for vaccination readiness.[30] The issues of vaccine delivery, distribution and administration were covered in this meeting. The states were informed that a single, national platform would be used to administer vaccines. The emergency use approval process was widely discussed. He directed the various regulators and experts in the room to ensure that the highest considerations of safety be taken into account while also observing what process the regulators of other key countries were following. The availability of the database of healthcare and frontline workers, augmentation of cold chains and procurement of syringes and needles were especially reviewed by the PM.

Soon after, PM Modi spoke to the CMs of all states,[31] explaining to them that India was on the verge of a big breakthrough. On 24 November, his message to the political leaders cutting party lines was clear. The vaccination programme was not just a government initiative, it was a national priority. There was no way to bounce back from the deep economic and social impact of the pandemic unless every state contributed and worked on the programme in mission mode.

The PM was very candid in explaining that the vaccination programme should not be looked at through a political lens. This effort needed not just a whole-of-government approach but also a whole-of-country approach. He talked about the four stages of the Indian psychological response to the pandemic. Initially, people were afraid of the virus, and it took some time for the mental models to transition from the first stage of fear to the second stage of doubts and exploration of information. Once people understood the virus better, their consciousness graduated to the third stage of acceptance. The fourth stage was negligence arising out of complacency about the virus.

The challenge to the vaccination process was that far too many people had crossed over to the territory of negligence. As the conditions had eased out, starting September, and the first wave had receded, people started to ignore the virus, assuming that no further damage would be inflicted by the invisible enemy. The PM cautioned the political leaders against this tendency that could lead to vaccine hesitancy or worse—indifference.

The states provided positive feedback on the ongoing efforts of the central government and resolved to work together on the vaccination programme. In a complex country like India, such interactions laying down a clear view of problems and potential solutions for a nationwide initiative were of the utmost importance. The success of the programme required political buy-in from all quarters. It was also critical that the message to the public at large was consistent, clear and positive.

The preparation between August and November set the stage for the decisive round. India's vaccination programme, the world's largest vaccination drive, was backed by carefully planned order and employed all the means the country had at its disposal.

National Vaccination Strategy

It was on 8 December 2020 that India unveiled the plan for what it had in store.[32] In a media interaction, Rajesh Bhushan, secretary, Ministry of Health and Family Welfare, outlined the key components of India's programme design.

Bhushan mentioned that the vaccination would be universal,

in that whoever wanted to take the vaccine would get it. Given the supply and demand mismatch, the vaccination programme would be launched in a phased manner. The first target was to cover 1 crore healthcare workers across public and private facilities, 2 crore frontline workers, which would include personnel from state and central police department, armed forces, home guard, civil defense organizations, disaster management volunteers and municipal workers, and about 30 crore others, who were over 50 years of age or had specific comorbidities.

Bhushan also confirmed the central government's intent to use the CoWIN platform, which stood for 'winning over Covid'. This platform was extrapolated from eVIN. The supply tracking and mediation platform was repurposed for demand tracking and fulfilment. This decision eventually proved to be a huge differentiator for how India accomplished the goal of vaccination saturation.

Bhushan also clarified that while there were 2.39 lakh vaccinators across India who participated in the UIP, only 1.54 lakh of these would be deployed for the Covid-19 vaccination. This was a tough decision, but it was necessary to ensure that regular vaccinations did not suffer. India had made hard-fought gains on infant and maternal mortality, progressively decreasing mortality rates. While Covid-19 was a huge public tragedy, the UIP, which competed for resources, network and human skill, could not be deprioritized for the Covid-19 vaccination. Both had to run in parallel and successfully. The government also committed to training more vaccinators, but the numbers would add up after a lag.

The NEGVAC also prescribed the presence of five vaccination officers at every centre. Each of these officers would be expected to play specific roles. There would be one vaccinator, an officer who is legally authorized to administer an injection. One officer would control the entry at the vaccination centre, checking all documents. A third officer would verify and authenticate all documents before vaccination. Two support officers would ensure crowd management and provide support to the vaccinator as required.

The strategy for choosing the first beneficiaries was based on the Values Framework of the SAGE of the WHO. Most countries followed this recommended approach. There were many debates within the NEGVAC on this question as well.

In one of the debates, a key official, who preferred not to be named, raised the question of vaccine hesitancy among the healthcare workers themselves. The WHO guideline on prioritizing the healthcare workers was well-intentioned. The intent was that the society reeling under the impact of the pandemic should not feel a dearth of healthcare workers. Once they acquired some immunity against the disease, their continuous availability would be a matter of great relief to society at large.

However, what was not envisaged were the opinions of the healthcare workers themselves. While this group was very vulnerable, it was also the group with the most amount of domain knowledge when it came to vaccines. There was a possibility that this group might be sceptical and would prefer to wait for more information on vaccines, not because they were against vaccines, but simply out of a desire to be well informed.

In the hotly debated NEGVAC meetings in December 2020, this question kept coming up. One view was regarding patient behaviour in India. Indians typically try to first seek peer validation on medical situations. They try to gather as much information as possible themselves through their own research and through friends and family. They approach the doctors with a loosely formulated view—right or wrong. The doctor may advise the opinion-seeker based on medical evidence. However, if the patient is not fully convinced, the typical approach is to ask the doctor, 'Doctor, what would you do if you were in my situation?'

One view in the NEGVAC meetings was that Covid-19 vaccines should not be subjected to this social consultation process. There had to be trust in the national regulators because if left to individual opinion—sometimes through social media-led public debates—it may lead to more doubts in the minds of those who did not understand the nuance. A doctor may try to explain that her personal comfort level was 9 on 10 and initiate a public debate for reasons of knowledge acquisition or dissemination. But what if the general public interpreted that as doctors not being fully sure?

Could there have been a different approach? Could India have employed a professional need-based vaccination strategy? For example, those in high-contact services—public transport, retail, hospitality, tourism sectors—could be vaccinated earlier. Several civil society organizations as well as think tanks had proposed various such strategies to the government. However, there was a risk of personal discretion in such approaches. If the guidelines were breached based on personal discretion, it could have become a national controversy and the process would have been compromised by acquiring political dimensions.

However, eventually, the NEGVAC came to the conclusion that the WHO guidelines should be followed. It was one of those decisions where the decision-makers knew there were many options with pluses and minuses. Yet, a decision had to be made in a firm manner, choosing only one option and overruling others.

The potential problem of vaccine hesitancy was, however, well recognized. The PM had already highlighted this problem to all the CMs on 24 November. His address had mentioned that there was a sense of complacency in the general population, which may have been a barrier for vaccine acceptance.

Building Trust in Indian Products: The PM's Personal Engagement

There was yet another aspect of vaccine acceptance that the PM wanted to address. The known vaccination efforts in India—be it polio or smallpox—had a 'foreign' element. It was generally assumed that vaccination against life-threatening diseases required a 'foreign hand' in controlling the vicissitudes these diseases inflicted. The PM decided to signal clearly and personally that the science and technology in India had to be trusted.

The PM decided to visit the Indian vaccine makers in a twofold manoeuvre.[33] His visit clearly put his weight behind the scientific efforts, thereby indicating to the government machinery that the vaccine makers had to be supported in whatever way was procedurally possible. The visit also told the country at large that India backed its scientists and research and development capabilities.

Around 8.00 a.m. on 28 November, the PM landed in Ahmedabad on an Indian Air Force (IAF) plane, from where he went to Changodar, the location of the Zydus Biotech Park, southeast of Ahmedabad. Pankaj Patel, the chairman of the firm, and his son, Sharvil Patel, managing director, welcomed the PM. Sharvil's wife, Meha, and their two young children were also part of the welcoming entourage. The PM spent a few moments with the children and then proceeded for the tour of the facility.

The Patels explained the work Zydus Cadila was broadly doing to combat Covid-19 as well as other diseases. They explained the unique DNA-based vaccine that their firm was developing, which was to be administered painlessly through an intradermal patch. Both the vaccine technology as well as the administration were different from other vaccine candidates. Finally, the PM, dressed in white-and-blue PPE, was given a tour of the manufacturing site.

Huge crowds had gathered outside the Zydus Biotech Park, aware of the PM's visit. He quickly waved to the waiting people and then proceeded to board his IAF flight to Hyderabad, which was the next stop. The flight landed at the Hakimpet Air Force base.

The PM proceeded to Shamirpet, the location of Hyderabad's Genome Valley, spread over an area of 600 sq. km. This large landscape, which hosts several companies working in the pharmaceutical as well as medical devices and related industries, was set up in 1999 as a PPP initiative. The chairman and managing director of Bharat Biotech, Dr Krishna Ella, was himself instrumental in setting up the Genome Valley on the outskirts of Hyderabad, northwest of the city. His son, Raches, and daughter-in-law, Sahari, welcomed the PM to the Bharat Biotech facility around 2.00 p.m.

The Bharat Biotech visit was critical because Covaxin was likely to be the first fully Indian vaccine to be deployed. Dr Krishna Ella and Suchithra Ella, the joint managing director, along with the members of the leadership team, briefed the PM, covering five broad areas. They started off by narrating the journey of the firm in the business of vaccines, especially talking about the rotavirus vaccine. Bharat Biotech's Rotavac completed 100 million doses worldwide, especially benefiting a lot of children in low- and middle-income countries. The Rotavac 5D vaccine, touted as the lowest dose volume vaccine, was launched by the firm in 2019, a bulwark against diarrhoea, a common problem for children, especially in poorer countries.

The Ellas then spoke about the development of Covaxin and their collaboration with the ICMR. They updated the PM on the progress of the vaccine development and expressed hope that the vaccine would be ready for rollout soon.

The next part of the briefing was focussed on the new nasal vaccine that Bharat Biotech was trialling. This intranasal vaccine targeted the virus in the nasal passage, thus preventing it from entering the lungs. The most severe form of Covid-19 was one when the virus attacked the lungs. The nasal vaccine focussed on early-stage prevention. Dr Krishna Ella requested support from the government on the development of this vaccine, as, in general, the testing protocols for such a technology were not robust. The government helped Bharat Biotech further this concept and permitted research on the vaccine, leading to a Phase II trial by August 2021. While eventually the focus shifted to Covaxin development, the nasal vaccine was not forgotten. By April 2022, the vaccine entered Phase III trials.[34] Eventually, India became one of the first countries to approve a nasal vaccine in September 2022.[35]

Dr Ella then informed the PM about the capacity constraints he faced at the Genome Valley in scaling up the production of Covaxin. Bharat Biotech could make about 1 crore doses a month at this facility. They had bigger capacity at their Bengaluru plant, which could be repurposed to produce 5 crore doses a month, but required quick approvals. Bharat Biotech was also willing to transfer technology to enable various public sector units around the country to make Covaxin.

All these requests were addressed by the government over the next few months. Bharat Biotech got an additional funding of ₹65 crore to scale up the Bengaluru plant.[36]

The last part of the briefing involved the PM interacting with the scientists at Bharat Biotech. He boosted their morale and urged them to work towards an effective indigenous vaccine with full dedication. The scientists also gave the PM a facility tour.

As he came out of the Bharat Biotech facility, the PM was again greeted by a welcoming crowd. He acknowledged them before boarding his black Toyota SUV. He left the Bharat Biotech site by 4.00 p.m. for Hakimpet and flew to Pune, his last stop for the day.

Pune is home to SII, established by Cyrus Poonawalla, chairman of the Poonawalla Group. The PM reached the SII on Solapur Road in the southeastern suburbs of Pune in a helicopter, a short 10-km ride from the main airport. He was received and welcomed by Cyrus Poonawalla, Adar Poonawalla, the CEO of the firm, and his wife Natasha, who is also the executive director of SII.

Adar proudly narrated the SII journey, which has been neatly inscribed on a big wall within the premises. This wall captures how the company has evolved, using its horse breeding experience to diversify in the business of vaccines.

The SII had already built a stockpile of more than 4 crore doses of Covishield at that point, fully expecting that the AstraZeneca trials would go smoothly and the vaccine would be approved. This was a big personal risk taken by the Poonawalla group, which demonstrated the commitment and true skin in the game Indian vaccine makers brought to the table.

Adar told the PM that SII would deliver 40 crore doses by July. The promise made by the young entrepreneur was to be fulfilled in due course as Covishield became the mainstay of the vaccination programme. The PM was then given a tour of the manufacturing facilities.

With the makeshift helipad not ready for late evening take-offs, the PM travelled back to the Pune airport in his car. He landed in New Delhi much behind the planned schedule. However, his visit had accomplished several things. The vaccine makers were reassured that the government was with them. The scientists in the three companies got a morale-boosting opportunity to interact with the PM. And people came to know about the great work being done by the Indian firms, thus setting the stage for better vaccine acceptance.

The PMO capped the evening with a press release:

> The scientists expressed joy that the Prime Minister met them face to face in order to boost their morale and help accelerate their efforts at this critical juncture in the vaccine development journey. The Prime Minister expressed pride in the fact that India's indigenous vaccine development has progressed at such a rapid pace so far. He spoke on how India is following sound principles of science in the entire journey of vaccine development, while also asking for suggestions to make the vaccine distribution process better.
>
> The Prime Minister stressed that India considers vaccines as not only vital to good health but also as a global good, and it is India's duty to assist other countries, including the nations in our neighborhood, in the collective fight against the virus.

> He asked the scientists to express their free and frank opinion on how the country could further improve its regulatory process. The scientists also presented an overview of how they are also developing various new and repurposed drugs to better fight COVID-19.[37]

From Laboratories to Arms

While the work on the vaccines was in full swing, a practical question to address was the adequate availability of supporting equipment required to store and administer vaccines. These included equipment like glass vials, glass tubes, rubber stoppers and syringes.

The vaccine makers were able to repurpose their assembly lines devoted to glass vials and associated equipment. But the vials still had to be made. This required increasing manufacturing capacity ahead of the vaccine availability. When the capital expenditure had to be made, it was not clear what size of glass vials would suffice for Covid-19 vaccines. Hence, new investment decisions had to be taken on a probabilistic basis. Several Indian firms rose to the occasion to expand their capacity right from mid-2020, anticipating the requirement down the line.[38]

On 27 April 2020, Rajiv Nath, managing director of the Hindustan Syringes and Medical Devices Limited, wrote[39] a letter to the secretary, Ministry of Health and Family Welfare. Nath stated that his firm was the largest manufacturer of auto-disable syringes in the country. These syringes were commonly used in India and he was willing to work on war footing to expand the syringe production capacity.

The government started buying syringes in preparation for the vaccination drive and creating a stockpile to ensure that no syringe shortage hit the country. This forward planning was very effective in ensuring that there were never any situations of syringe shortages at the vaccination centres.

Nath's firm started supplying syringes to the government in December 2020 and eventually delivered 820 million auto-disable syringes to the government in the next 20 months. Additionally, his firm supplied 565 million syringes to international clients, like UNICEF and Pan American Health Organization. Countries like Japan and Brazil also relied on his firm. Eventually, his firm delivered 1.6 billion syringes of various types and capacities in 20 months, till August 2022.[40]

While this is the story of one firm, it shows the strength of Make in India and the extent of forward preparedness different stakeholders brought to the table. While, over the course of the vaccination drive, these elements were taken for granted in India, it was not the case around the world. Several countries had to scramble to arrange syringes.[41]

On part of the Indian government, the lockdown rules in 2020 made adequate provisions for the manufacturing sector. The manufacturing sector focussing on pharmaceutical goods was permitted to remain open following all Covid-19 protocols. This was an important part of the planning because the required capacity expansion had to be done significantly ahead of the vaccine availability. While in 2020 fighting the pandemic was the obvious problem on everyone's mind, the public and the private sector was working together to prepare for what lay ahead.

From the equipment required to fight the pandemic, like masks, sanitizers, PPE kits and medicines to equipment that may be required in the future for vaccination, India ramped up production capacity for this broad range throughout 2020. The lockdown rules had to be specifically tailored for such a ramp-up based on industry requirement.

Communication Planning

The government machinery was already working on a comprehensive communication plan to ensure that Indians were comforted about the vaccine and all their questions were answered. One of the key inputs to this communication effort was the learning from India's polio vaccination programme.[42] It was clear that rapidly dispelling misinformation and addressing all rumours head-on, strongly and unambiguously was the key to building trust and confidence in vaccines in society.

The Ministry of Health and Family Welfare released a detailed communication strategy to be used at central, state and district levels. This was authored by in-house experts as well as external consultants who had experience working in the social sector. Padmaja Singh, joint secretary in the ministry, Dr Veena Dhawan, official in the Immunization Division of the ministry, and Gauri Rishi, social and behaviour change consultant, were instrumental in putting this document together.[43] Experts from UNICEF, BMGF and the Immunization Technical Support Unit of the ministry provided valuable support and inputs.

The document focussed on addressing not just vaccine hesitancy but also vaccine eagerness and the importance of following Covid-19 appropriate behaviour even after vaccination. It also outlined the role of the media, social media and the need for quickly addressing any adverse effects of vaccination to retain trust in the vaccines.

Speaking at the foundation stone laying ceremony of AIIMS at Rajkot in Gujarat, PM Modi expressed confidence that India was ready to start the mass vaccination programme soon.[44] The last day of the year ended on a cautiously optimistic note.

The annus horribilis was drawing to a close. As much as the country had suffered, the public attention and discourse were now focussed on how quickly the jabs would make it to the Indian arms.

9

THE VACCINES ROLL OUT

India started the vaccination roll-out targeting the healthcare workers and frontline workers as the first set of recipients. In a well-considered strategy after weighing the pros and cons of this approach, India stuck to the similar norms being used internationally.

On 16 January, PM Narendra Modi kicked off the vaccination drive through a video conference at 10.30 a.m.[1] More than 3,000 vaccination sites were connected through the video conference for this event, with each site expected to run one session with a capacity of up to 100 jabs to be administered.

India aimed to vaccinate 3 crore high-risk professionals in the opening round. This was to be followed by opening up the vaccination programme for 30 crore individuals identified on the basis of age and risk perception for the virus.

Speaking at the launch event, the PM noted that 3 crore itself was a big number in the global context, being more than the population of a 100 countries.[2] This also contextualized the challenges that lay ahead for India, simply in terms of the numbers. He reiterated that people should not pay heed to rumours and believe in the talent and competence of Indian scientists and researchers.[3] This message was critical to addressing potential hesitancy and acceptance issues and was repeated in various ways through the next few months.

PM Modi announced this drive through his Twitter feed, sharing a short video with the theme—'*Sarve bhavantu sukhinah,*

Sarve santu niramayah', a Sanskrit verse meaning 'May all be happy, may all be free of illnesses.' His tweet read: 'India begins the world's #LargestVaccineDrive. This is a day of pride, a celebration of the prowess of our scientists and hard work of our medical fraternity, nursing staff, police personnel and sanitation workers. May everyone be healthy and free from illness.'[4]

The vaccination programme was to be a free exercise in the government centres. India budgeted a massive ₹35,000 crore or $4.65 billion in the Union Budget for the financial year 2021–22 for this exercise. This was a big cost to the public exchequer, but it was important to not burden the society with the costs of the vaccines. The cost to the economy by not vaccinating enough number of people would have been significantly higher.

On the first day of the vaccination drive, a total of 3,352 sessions were held, in which 191,181 beneficiaries were vaccinated.[5] A total of 16,755 personnel were actively involved in the massive nationwide vaccination roll-out.

India started tracking AEFI right from the first day. In fact, the vaccinations were rolled out with a standard process that the recipient of the jab would have to wait for 30 minutes at the vaccination site under observation. This would help in spotting any potential health issues and getting adequate medical attention.

In the initial weeks, each state scheduled Covid-19 vaccination for four days a week, retaining the other days for other vaccinations. This gradual phase-in was required to ensure that existing immunization programmes were not disturbed for lack of vaccinators. This approach also gave states the time to familiarize themselves with how the process of vaccination worked, including better understanding of the vaccine supply chain, movement and its fine-tuning as more data and insights became available.

The first 1 crore or 10 million doses were administered by 19 February 2021.[6] It took India 34 days to hit this critical milestone.

Expanding the Programme

On 28 February, during the last weekend of the month, the CoWIN platform was upgraded to CoWIN 2.0.[7] This change formed the backbone of the first major scale-up of the vaccination programme.

The government announced that starting 1 March, all Indians who were more than 60 years of age or who were 45 years of age and had any of the 20 specified comorbidities would be eligible to get a vaccine dose.[8]

With the healthcare workers and frontline workers covered adequately, the idea was to move to the next most at-risk population cohort. The appointments were to be booked via CoWIN, and once the person got an appointment, they could go to the specified centre and get the vaccine dose.

At this time, both SII as well as Bharat Biotech were just beginning to expand their manufacturing capacity. But the numbers at this time were only gradually building up. By the end of February, India had administered 1.34 crore or 13.4 million doses. This number rose to 6.43 crore or 64.3 million by the end of March. About 5 crore or 50 million doses were administered in that month.[9]

While the progress was slow relative to the size of the Indian population, there were early signs that month-on-month growth of vaccination numbers would be strong. However, looking at these numbers in isolation, it would appear that India was a long way away from getting anywhere close to covering the whole country. While such analysis is simplistic, it is always easy to look at specific data and then assume that real world data moves linearly. The early euphoria regarding vaccination began to grow hazy with doubts being cast and criticism mounting.

'Tell someone that everything will be great and they're likely to either shrug you off or offer a sceptical eye. Tell someone they're in danger and you have their undivided attention.'[10] This theory worked perfectly during pandemic times. While public policy and governance are enriched by informed criticism, the operative word is 'informed'. To say that India is administering 5 crore vaccine doses a month but it should instead be doing 50 crore doses a month would not be informed criticism. It would simply be an opinion, which of course anyone would be free to hold, but it would not add any value to public discourse.

Unfortunately, a lot of criticism at that time focussed on such polemics rather than understanding the multivariate problem at hand.

'India Would Take a Decade to Vaccinate'

Of all the criticism that emerged in March–April 2021, the most surreal was a simple Excel sheet-based extrapolation of vaccine doses delivered into the future. Essentially, analysts myopically took the number of vaccine doses administered in some month or an average of the dose count in one or two months and simply extrapolated that on to the Indian population. India's total population was divided with the average number of vaccinations being administered a month and inferred that India may take years or even a decade to vaccinate its entire population.

Such extrapolation was also done in 2020 by some individuals, who projected that a significant part of the Indian population would be infected with Covid-19 by the second or the third quarter of that year.[11]

'India will take 12 years to vaccinate entire population, reach herd immunity in 8 years at current pace,' a report said.[12] This was not an isolated instance of this perspective. Such literature was commonplace in these months. The media and social media frenzy fed into each other. It was difficult to establish how this analysis perpetuated. However, many people believed such articles, tweets and WhatsApp forwards, which led to building a wall of negativity.

In the end, of course, such criticism was to be proven childish.

The real India performed significantly better than Excel sheet derivations, it also did better than reasonable-sized 'reference countries', which were being quoted as contrasting examples in the early months.

'The Government Should Have Given More Money to Vaccine Makers'

Another common critique of the government was that India should have pumped in more money for the two primary vaccine markers in these initial months, so that they could have been better equipped to handle a massive scale-up of production.

This thinking comes from the conventional process of manufacturing industries, where the product is produced in big quantities and the capital expenditure and production quantity are directly related. If a company makes X tonnes of cement by investing an amount N, it can create a second plant by putting in the same amount, whereby 2N would produce 2X quantity of the cement—double the original. These are the types of assumptions used for industry and company analysis and, of course, they work in a certain context.

But for discrete manufacturing, where the end product is produced in batches, such linear extrapolation does not always work. If a car manufacturer produces 100 cars a month in one factory, can they naturally produce 200 cars a month if they invest in a second identical factory? This is where process manufacturing differs from discrete manufacturing. In the case of the latter, the process is well standardized, but a new assembly line may have its own unique problems. It may take some time to stabilize a new facility or line.

This was empirically validated from examples outside India, too. As we now know from the experience of the western vaccine makers, throwing more money at the vaccine lines did not necessarily scale up their capacity exponentially. Putting in advance orders did not mean anything—as the EU learnt the hard way. When the Indian government was fending off criticism about vaccine manufacturing not scaling up, those interested in getting vaccinated were being forced to wait for weeks in several countries in Europe. The advance orders placed by the EU in 2020 did not fully materialize until the later part of April 2021.

A more realistic criticism could have been that the government could have funded the vaccine makers' expansion earlier than it did. On 19 April 2021, the government approved[13] ₹3,000 crore (nearly $40 million) for SII to invest in expansion. As soon as the new financial year kicked in on 1 April, this decision was put in motion.

Could the government have done this a month earlier and if yes, what impact would it have had on quantities of vaccine production? It is unclear if the decision taken on 19 April had any negative impact. The SII embraced at-risk production at a much more delicate stage using its internal accruals. Would this have been a decision with extraordinarily high marginal utility, cutting a few months from the eventual time it took for vaccine coverage? There is no compelling counterfactual to establish along these lines.

'The Second Wave Could Have Been Prevented by Vaccines'

India saw a devastating second wave of Covid-19 in April and May 2021. The infection count started to rise towards the end of February, but the rise was not steep until late March. However, starting late March, things took a turn for the worse. India entered April clocking about 80,000 daily Covid-19 cases and exited April with a daily count of almost 400,000 cases.

This kind of a rise in daily cases could have overwhelmed any healthcare system around the world. To top it, the Delta variant was significantly more lethal than its predecessors. The country faced a grim situation with a mounting death toll and a general sense of helplessness against the brutal pathogen.

In April, there was a theory that the second wave was quite ferocious in India because the country had been slow in vaccinating its people. There is, of course, nothing to take away from the human tragedy endured by families around India. However, it would be disingenuous to say that a bigger number of vaccinations between January and March would have prevented this tragedy.

For example, the US, which started its vaccination programme on 13 December 2020, a month before India, had administered 10.86 crore or 108.6 million doses till 31 March 2021.[14] If the US, with captive access to vaccines and its influence over vaccine makers, could not cover the country in three-and-a-half months, could India have done that in two-and-a-half months?

Working backwards from 1 April, knowing that India was to separate the two doses by 28 days and assuming that it took two weeks for the antibodies to build up, nationwide coverage would only be possible by completing the administration of second doses by mid-March. This would mean that nationwide administration of the first dose would have to be completed by mid-February. Clearly, this was a theoretical argument.

To top it off, vaccine hesitancy was a non-trivial factor in February and March, when the vaccination rate built up gradually.

There are many lessons for India to learn from the second wave of the pandemic with respect to its healthcare system. But that the second wave happened due to poor vaccine coverage is not an argument that holds ground.

'The Private Sector Should Have Been Involved Earlier'

India's healthcare systems are bimodal—the public sector and the private sector work side-by-side, sometimes performing overlapping functions and sometimes carrying out exclusively assigned tasks. There was no doubt that the private sector had to be engaged at some point to make the vaccination effort successful.

When the vaccination started in January, the government kicked off the process in the public sector. State governments and, through them, municipal and local bodies, were engaged to undertake this exercise. This mirrored the three-tier public healthcare architecture.

There were suggestions in the initial weeks that the government should have involved the private sector upfront in the process. If this had been done right at the inception, there would have been the challenge of keeping the vaccination programme truly equitable. Large private players, such as corporate hospitals, would have accessed disproportionately high quantities of vaccines and administered them at a price.

In fact, when the private sector was eventually allowed, this scenario[15] did play out in some parts of the country. If, in the early period of the vaccination drive, government decisions would have created a perception of vaccine inequity, it would have deeply impacted the acceptance of the vaccines themselves. The poor would have seen the drive as a multi-speed programme, with express exclusion of those who could not afford to pay.

'The government should allow those who can pay' may sound like a good argument when made by those who can pay. But it would have had devastating consequences for those who couldn't. Ultimately, the government phased in private sector participation with a targeted role.

'Allow Anyone to Procure'

The vaccination programme was devised in a way that the central government would place orders and then apportion the quantities received to the state governments, which would then send the vaccines onwards to districts, which were controlling the end destination—hospitals, CHCs and PHCs.

As the vaccination numbers moved modestly to 5 crore in

the month of April, another criticism gained ground. Pressure built up on the government to end its procurement monopoly. There were arguments that the central government should not be the only entity procuring vaccines. State governments should also be allowed to procure them.

This argument was based on two assumptions. First, the central government was not able to procure large quantities of vaccines because it was doing something wrong. Second, by letting the states procure vaccines directly, the process would become efficient, equitable and representative of true federal democracy.

Neither were reasonable arguments—the world of vaccines was simply production-constrained. Even if India were to negotiate with a Pfizer or a Moderna for getting vaccines, would it be better for the country to negotiate as a whole or allow states to bargain for smaller quantities going head-to-head against each other? The answer must have been clear to anyone who remotely understands the economics of scale and commercial contracting.

This was also the time when the second wave of Covid-19 was hurting the country badly. The states also wanted a greater role for themselves in making the vaccines available.

Historically, all major vaccination efforts in India have been nationally driven, such as the EPI, launched in 1978, and the Pulse Polio Programme. However, given that the states had a crucial role to play in managing the pandemic, they increasingly felt the need to take matters into their own hands during the Delta wave.

The central government made significant changes to the vaccination programme on 19 April 2021, giving a chance to the states to make their arguments work on the ground. It opened up not just the vaccine eligibility conditions, it also allowed multi-sourced supply. In essence, both the demand and the supply side were liberalized.

A New Procurement Approach

The central government made several far-reaching announcements on 19 April.[16]

The pricing, procurement, eligibility and administration of vaccines were made totally flexible starting 1 May 2021. The national vaccination drive was opened to everyone who was 18 years of age or above. The vaccine manufacturers were incentivized to further scale up their production and foreign manufacturers were permitted to bid for Indian contracts.

The central government also gave up its monopoly of local procurement. It allowed vaccine manufacturers to release up to 50 per cent of their supply to the states and also to the open markets—private hospitals—at a pre-declared price. The new directive ensured that the states did not have any price disadvantage over the central government when buying from the local manufacturers.

The states were empowered to procure additional vaccine doses directly from the manufacturers, as well as to open up vaccination to any category of people above the age of 18 as they deemed fit in their jurisdiction. The central government-sponsored vaccination drive was to continue as before, providing free vaccination for essential and priority populations.

This change gave a sense of self-actualization to the critics of the extant policies. Commentators hailed the central government for these measures but also claimed credit for having forced the central government into 'doing the right thing'.

States got ready to float their tenders. In fact, many municipal bodies also got ready to attract foreign vaccine makers. All along, the operating assumption was that because India had not floated public tenders for Covid-19 vaccines, there was a countrywide shortage.

Experience Holds a Dear School

The opening up of vaccinations for all Indian adults led to an initial euphoria. Starting 1 May, CoWIN slot bookings became a prized asset. As the slots for vaccination opened every night, millions of Indians would log in to the platform. While some would be successful, others not. The reason was clear—the vaccine production quantities were moving up, but gradually.

However, the states were upbeat about their ability to buy vaccines. Tenders were floated by various public bodies in early May, with the hope that vaccine makers would come rushing in with miraculously high quantities of supply. This process had unintended consequences.

Domestic vaccine makers started being pressured by politicians across states to accord them priority for vaccine supply. When the central government was the sole procurer, it routed predetermined quantities to each state. No state would have been happy with the supplies of a limited commodity they received. However, there was a logic and rationale in such allocation.

Even if states or their residents were unhappy, the central government took the blame, acting as a backstop. While the central government was working with a plan, states were accusing it of being partial or arbitrary in its vaccine allocation. They thought they could do a better job.

As soon as the changed policy was announced on 19 April, there was a clamour to influence the vaccine makers. In just two weeks, the situation became so grim that Adar Poonawalla, the CEO of the SII had to leave Pune for London for safety measures. He stated that he had started getting threatening calls[17] for prioritizing supplies to specific states. The situation got so vitiated almost immediately that the SII even announced[18] a fresh investment in the UK for vaccine expansion.

While, as a private entity, the SII was free to make its own investment calls, it was a poignant moment. In just two weeks,

India's flagship vaccine maker faced so much political pressure that it was forced to consider alternative geographical expansion. This was a sad moment, especially because the SII had been committed to Pune as their preferred business destination for decades. The hard and soft investments the group made over the decades had reached their breaking point in just two weeks.

The states continued to push their agenda of tenders with a view that they could do something better than the central government. It took just about four weeks for the penny to drop.

Maharashtra, India's most industrial and amongst the richest states, drew a blank on its tenders. In Mumbai, the local municipal body's global tender for vaccines was a flop, with all nine bids junked due to one or the other inadequacy.[19]

On 25 May, a *Times of India* report stated: 'Many states across the country have floated global tenders for procuring vaccines. But they have not yielded any results because of shortage of doses and other licences required, said another health official. Many states have now turned to the Centre to float global tender for procuring vaccines, which would benefit the states in turn.'[20]

In just four weeks, the states wanted the Centre to take back the procurement control, something they had fought to get for several months. By early June, the worst effects of the Delta wave were beginning to recede as well. At this point, the states realized that the vaccination drive, along with the credit and blame that came with it, was best left for the central government to handle. The appetite for decentralized procurement waned suddenly.

Back on Track

PM Modi made a televised address to the nation on 7 June, reversing a short-lived vaccine procurement policy stance. India reverted to the old system of procurement with some other tweaks to the design of vaccine administration.

In his address, the PM said:

After much deliberation, it was agreed that if the state governments also want to make efforts on their behalf, so why should the Indian government object? In view of this demand from the states and keeping in mind their request, a change was made in the system which was going on since January 16 as an experiment. We thought that when the states are making this demand and they have enthusiasm, let's give 25 percent of the work to them. As a result, 25 percent of the work was handed over to the states from May 1 and they also made efforts in their own way to complete it. [...]

Today it has been decided that the Government of India will also bear the responsibility of 25 percent of the work related to vaccination with the states. This arrangement will be implemented in the next two weeks. In these two weeks, the central and state governments together will make necessary preparations according to the new guidelines. Coincidentally, two weeks later, International Yoga Day falls on June 21. From June 21, the Government of India will provide free vaccines to the states for all citizens above the age of 18 years. The Government of India itself will buy 75 per cent of the total vaccine production from vaccine manufacturers and give it to the state governments free of cost. That is, no state government of the country will have to spend anything on the vaccine. Till now, crores of people of the country have got free vaccines.

Now people of 18 years of age will also become part of it. Only the Government of India will provide free vaccines to all the countrymen. Whether it is poor, lower middle class, middle class, or upper class, only the free vaccines will be administered in the Government of India campaign. Those who do not want to get the vaccine for free and want to get the vaccine in a private hospital have also been taken care of. The system of private sector hospitals procuring 25 percent

> of the vaccine being made in the country will continue. Private hospitals will be able to charge a maximum service charge of Rs 150 for a single dose after the prescribed price of the vaccine. The task of monitoring it will remain with the state governments.[21]

The states gladly accepted the change, though it would have been better if the original plan had been maintained. Notably absent from the scene were the vocal critics who had advocated decentralized procurement in April.

After 21 June 2021, India did not look back.

10

VACCINE JUGGERNAUT: LORD JAGANNATHA'S IRRESISTIBLE FORCE REPLAYED

Six months into 2021, all of India had been through a rollercoaster of emotions with respect to Covid-19. Apprehension gave way to utter despair during the depths of the Delta wave and progressed to general wariness and then a glimmer of hope. Halfway into the year, there was no guarantee that things would improve, and no one was confident enough to think the worst was already well behind.

Yet, humans, as prone as they are to their own personal weaknesses, shortcomings and drawbacks, are fundamentally resilient creatures. Beyond our petty squabbles and divisions, our fundamental instinct remains a positive desire for our collective stability and well-being, and the willingness to recognize and align behind such efforts.

The Exponential Curves Start Showing Up

Announcements, such as the central government's decision to resume vaccine procurement, are themselves not a source of credibility. However, *data* is. A few were keeping a close eye on the daily vaccination and supply figures that the Ministry of Health and Family Welfare was diligently reporting every day. The data was telling.

April saw a substantial 9 crore or 90 million vaccinations.

Through the end of April and throughout May, as states and the Centre, along with private players, contended for vaccines, supply and distribution were constrained, with total vaccinations falling to 6 crore or 60 million that month.

Since April 2021, the SII had been working to expand the monthly production to 10 crore or 100 million doses. During the month of June, it successfully scaled up production yield above 10 crore or 100 million doses for the first time.[1]

Those keenly following the vaccine production and administration data would have noted the consistent supply of vaccines since the beginning of June. The first week of June saw nearly 2 crore or 20 million doses, already a third of the month of May. The second week saw 2.2 crore or 22 million doses. The third week saw almost 2.5 crore or 25 million doses administered, keeping up the rising trend. The fourth week saw a colossal 4.5 crore or 45 million jabs. The entire month of June would see 12.3 crore or 123 million vaccinations—by far the highest up to that point.[2] This was equivalent to vaccinating all citizens of the world's twelfth largest country at least once.

The authors' analysis of this data continuously reinforced the statements coming from both major vaccine makers—their yields were stable or rising in June, and the gap between their early monthly estimates and actual delivered volumes was falling. This was a clear sign that they were gaining better control over scaling their production process. The supply and consumption data through the month bore this out.

Surprisingly though, this was nearly entirely ignored by the mainstream media, which was almost completely bereft of any substantial analysis of detailed production and consumption data. The authors reported on this topic in clinical detail in early June 2021.[3] This article published in *Swarajya* magazine noted:

> The latest data indicates the difficult period of vaccine supply, and demand imbalance is now nearly past. The

> strong increase in vaccination numbers for the past two and half weeks aligns closely with the statements made by the vaccine manufacturers that supply would rise by the end of May. From 250 million by the end of this week, India will probably see over 300 million doses consumed by the end of the month.

All of this turned out to be accurate—three weeks after that article, June ended with India producing a cumulative 328 million vaccines. It turned out to be the best-performing month until then. That it was also the worst-performing month when compared to every single month of the second half of 2021 showed how India's vaccination programme grew exponentially.

TABLE 8

Month-Wise Vaccine Doses Administered[4]

Month	*Vaccines Administered (million doses)*
June 2021	123.8
July 2021	127.7
August 2021	183.9
September 2021	238.9
October 2021	171.2
November 2021	177.3
December 2021	210.7

The authors have long contended that the positive direction of the Indian vaccination effort was visible quite early in the vaccine production data trends. The authors worked with a combination of two data points—the statements made by the vaccine producers and the daily actual consumption data available that was being patiently accumulated and analysed.

Making a clean break from the tenor of public discourse that sought to back or discredit the governments either at the central or state levels, this quantitative effort ignored that debate entirely; it sought to focus entirely on the numbers. The raw numbers gave credence to the statements of the producers. They enabled the extrapolation of future performance estimates, which could be successively validated week after week.

Both the key manufacturers, SII and Bharat Biotech, continued to put out important statistics in the public domain. Sometimes they were criticized for going overboard in almost a marketing-like effort. But it can be safely concluded in hindsight that even if some statements may have been put out a few weeks in advance, it was only a few weeks until the actual output caught up. The portrayal of Indian manufacturing was not empty rhetoric—it was backed by rapidly adjusting and increasing vaccine quantities.

Several weeks of relentless effort in this manner yielded a consistent picture of production estimates being met, which, in turn, offered a greater level of confidence in the forward-looking statements being made by the manufacturers.

It was not simply a question of choosing whom to believe. It started from the 'source of truth', the vaccine producers, and attempted to validate their estimates against visible vaccine consumption data over a period of time. There's admittedly very little excitement in this; it involved updating published data every single day for weeks, cross-referencing against statements made by vaccine makers and establishing how close the estimates and reality were.

As early as the second week of April, this analysis yielded the risk of a supply problem[5] that would later be seen between the end of April and the end of May. It recommended the administration of first doses in the third week of April.[6] In fact on 17 May, the government did change the gap between the two doses of Covishield to 84 days.[7]

This decision was also questioned, but, again, the passage of time has shown that Indian vaccination timing helped in mitigating the severity of the third or fourth wave, which were significantly milder than those in the other parts of the world and definitely milder than the first two waves of the pandemic in the country.

Similarly, data correctly showed that there was limited benefit in following the West in making bulk pre-orders—India, in fact, chose its own, far more effective procurement mechanism.[8]

While all of this raw data was readily accessible to the public, it was unfortunate that mainstream media did not make the effort to parse it to offer the Indian public a more nuanced, data-driven understanding of the situation related to India's vaccination efforts. Had the data been analysed better, several consequent realities would have been apparent weeks or months in advance. For example, it was clear from the rapid vaccine consumption in early April due to the Delta wave that there would be a domino effect later that month and in May, resulting in a shortage, as production yields had not risen sufficiently at that time.

Covishield started from a stable production rate of 40–50 million doses in early 2021, scaled up to 60–70 million doses around May, 100 million in June, 120 million in July and 150 million in August. In doing so, it was outproducing almost every other major vaccine in production and was one of the top three produced vaccines in the world, along with Sinovac and Pfizer/BioNTech, both of which were backed by far more economically powerful nations.

The Juggernaut

Even amidst the national carnage of the second wave, which peaked in May, where national resources were commandeered to transport oxygen and life-saving medical supplies across the country, the ongoing vaccinations happening in the middle of that calamity were impressive.

TABLE 9

Top Three Countries: Cumulative Vaccinations up to 30 April 2021[9]

Country	*Vaccines Administered (million doses)*
China	265
US	262
India	152

TABLE 10

Top Three Countries: Total Vaccinations in April 2021[10]

Country	*Vaccines Administered (million doses)*
China	145
US	90
India	87

As much as the end of April 2021 was a period no Indian would like to relive, history records the following reality. The very nadir of the Covid-19 situation in India, April 2021, was also the last month India ranked below the second position in the cumulative number of vaccinations.

As the second most populous country, this had to be a given—India was bound to occupy the first or second position in such a ranking as a baseline requirement. The reality is that by the end of April, it did. More importantly, it did so *on its own*. Barring about a million imported doses of Sputnik V vaccine, forming just 0.05 per cent of the 2 billion vaccine doses administered,[11] this programme was driven by domestic capability.

North America and Western Europe called upon an array of

multinational production sites across their geographical extent, with the initially low US production being compensated by an early surge in EU production, which the US imported. As a combination of vaccine production problems and politically driven vaccine hesitancy hit the latter, India overtook the US in May to finish as the nation with the second-highest number of vaccinations, behind China.

In June, India far outstripped the US and overtook the entire combined EU vaccination count. In July, India proceeded to far outstrip the EU and almost caught up with the combined vaccinations of the entire continent of Europe—the EU, the British Isles and every other European nation together.

By August 2021, India far exceeded the entire western developed world, all of Europe and all of North America combined. It reached the zenith in September 2021, when vaccinations in India exceeded the combined vaccinations of Europe, North America, South America and Africa, hitting almost 240 million vaccinations in that month alone. That is a sustained average of nearly 8 million people vaccinated every single day, all month long.

By the last quarter of 2021, India proceeded to overtake China's monthly vaccination rate. In each of the third and fourth calendar quarters of 2021, India administered half a billion vaccinations, a daily average of more than 6 million—a number more than the populations of Denmark, Singapore or New Zealand—per day across over half a year.

At the end of 2021, over 1.45 billion vaccine doses, including first and second doses, had been administered in India, a cumulative figure more than the total population. Till 15 January 2022, one year from when the vaccination programme started in 2021, India saw 1.57 billion vaccinations, a full-year average vaccination rate of a colossal 43 lakh or 4.3 million vaccinations a day.[12]

These are just a small set of the array of statistics on what ensued in the immediate aftermath of the second wave. But this is not an exercise in triumphalist deflection.

What Transpired?

Between 1 July and 31 December 2021, a total of 112 crore or 1.12 billion vaccinations were administered in India in 182 days. The mathematical average rate here is trivial to compute but astounding to contemplate—every single day of that half-year period saw 61.5 lakh or 6.15 million vaccines being administered.

To appreciate the size of that number and the effort it takes to sustain such a high average vaccination rate over such a long period, it is worth considering the populations of some major cities. Ahmedabad has a population of 6.3 million. Chennai city, not the whole metropolis, has fewer than 5 million people. Denmark, Norway, Singapore and New Zealand have population of approximately 6.15 million each.

As a comparative benchmark, to date, each of these countries have vaccinated between 80 and 92 per cent of their population with at least one dose cumulatively since the vaccinations started. India achieved this feat every single day on an average for six months straight. India did more in one day for 182 days at a stretch than some of the richer countries did in a whole year.

The Indian government deserves all the credit for the success of this effort. It is easy for vaccination efforts to stall at critical moments. North America saw its share of population that had at least one dose rise just seven percentage points from 68 per cent to 75 per cent in the first half of 2022.[13] India saw the same figure increase from 61 per cent to 73 per cent in the same period, exceeding all of North America (the combined US, Canada and Mexico) in the process—three times as much—though India's population is 2.3 times the population of North America.

India's state capacity, not often recognized, let alone feted, rose to the occasion, day after day, across the country.

11

CELEBRATING PM MODI'S BIRTHDAY IN STYLE

If the number of people receiving a vaccine dose in India alone on 17 September 2021 formed a country, it would be the fifty-sixth largest country[1] in the world.

PM Narendra Modi was born on 17 September 1950. On his birthday in 2021, the Indian Covid-19 vaccination programme was in full swing. India administered 2.5 crore or 25 million vaccine doses on this day.[2] This was like vaccinating the entire population of Australia once in a single day.

As many as 2.5 crore vaccines in a day translated to 10.42 lakh or 1.04 million vaccines per hour, 17,360 doses per minute or 289 doses per second. These are the average numbers over a day, but the peak hours were significantly higher. Every state in the country worked in mission mode on this day to bring forth the true inherent capacity of the Indian healthcare sector. CoWIN, the backbone of this system, worked flawlessly despite the high user activity and simultaneous logins from around India.

Linking Commemorative Day to Social Service

It is customary in the Indian political landscape for party functionaries to celebrate their leaders' birthdays in ways that enable them to reach large sections of society. Such occasions are commonly used by political functionaries to increase their own visibility as well as propagate their party's message to citizens at large.

On 17 September, similarly, a campaign titled 'Vaccine Seva' was run by many individuals around India to mark PM Modi's birthday. This campaign was different from the usual political activities, as it was directly linked to a greater good at a crucial time. Volunteers around the country helped vaccine seekers by registering them on the CoWIN app and assisted them with access to the vaccination centres.

To take the campaign to a broad section of people, a social media campaign identified by the hashtag #VaccineSeva was also run. This further amplified the message and helped enrol more volunteers around the country. Politicians travelled to various parts of the country to oversee the proceedings, also amplifying messages of Vaccine Seva.

Health Minister Mansukh Mandaviya encouraged these efforts personally. He shared the #VaccineSeva tweets of Nishant[3] from Pune and Ankita Sood[4] from Mumbai to highlight some personal contributions from this unique campaign, furthering a national cause.

Numbers Add Up

With the registrations for vaccination swelling and each state rushing to add more, India crossed 1 crore or 10 million doses by 1.30 p.m., 2 crore or 20 million doses just after 5.00 p.m. and then, eventually, 2.5 crore or 25 million doses around midnight.[5]

The previous highest single day vaccination figure of 1.33 crore or 13.3 million doses was surpassed easily and nearly doubled on 17 September.

This single-day surge also took India's total vaccine coverage past the 80-crore or 800-million mark. The journey from 70 crore to 80 crore, or 700 million to 800 million, was covered merely in 11 days.

The first 10 crore or 100 million doses came in 45 days. The the next six additional 10 crore doses took 29, 24, 20, 19 and 13 days, respectively. And then, the 17 September surge meant that the eight blocks of 10 core doses were administered in just 11 days.[6]

This progression was a testament to the fact that India had been learning from the past experience rapidly and tweaking systems and processes to speed up the vaccination process. It also demonstrated that the vaccine manufacturing had picked up pace.

Logistics behind the Record

India did not reach the 2.5 crore or 25 million single-day vaccination mark coincidentally. Significant planning went into the canvassing that happened across the country.

The volunteer networks treated this exercise similar to how they would treat an election day task. Indian general elections lead to the biggest mobilization of humanity in the world, with the election machinery working like clockwork.

Political actors manage the election day process through the knowledge of booths and electoral roll. The booth-level volunteers are required to 'get the vote out' in the micro-segments of villages, towns and cities assigned to them. This process has been learnt and perfected by those associated with the political spectrum.

This same process was followed on 17 September, with similar mobilization efforts made for the vaccine drive. Volunteers knew exactly how to go door-to-door and were often known to the residents they were about to approach.

The demand for the vaccines had to be matched with the supply as well. This was also the time vaccine availability in India had begun to improve at a rapid pace with both SII and Bharat Biotech being able to ramp up production. The month of September 2021 had already seen the administration of an average of 75 lakh or 7.5 million vaccine doses per day. The states were well equipped with the increasing number of doses available from both the leading manufacturers. As of 16 September, with 1.65 crore or 16.5 million doses in the pipeline, the states already had an inventory of 5.3 crore or 53 million doses of the vaccines.[7]

Hence, an ideal demand and supply match was available in this timeframe, with the number of vaccinators and sessions possible being the limiting factor. Ultimately, the 2.5-crore or 25-million mark was achieved with what is called 'full-court press' in the game of basketball.

At least eight states—Assam, Bihar, Gujarat, Karnataka, Madhya Pradesh, Rajasthan, Telangana and Uttarakhand set new records for highest single-day vaccinations on 17 September.[8] There were other local initiatives also undertaken on this day. For example, in Mumbai, the local civic body organized special camps for vaccinating women.[9]

Mandaviya personally supervised the day's proceedings, not leaving his office until the wee hours of the morning on 18 September. He worked with his teams through the day to ensure that there were no vaccine logistics issues anywhere in the country. He also monitored the numerical progress on an hourly basis, using his Twitter feed to update the country as numbers kept adding. Finally, after a long day, he made sure that the numbers from states were tallied properly and authentically.[10]

The entire process brought together the age-old technique of using an episodic push for public health programmes. This technique has been used in India for pulse polio campaigns too, where specifically earmarked days saw a surge of vaccine coverage. This entire vaccination machinery can coalesce with known and specific targets to meet the goal on the stated day.

Prime Minister's Response

Speaking at an event in Goa through video conference on 18 September, PM Modi remarked, 'With your efforts, India has created a world record of administering over 2.5 crore vaccines in a single day, a feat not even the most powerful nations have been able to achieve.'[11]

September 2021 was the turning point for the Indian vaccine coverage. Practically all possible doubts and questions that were raised in the previous six months were answered. The creases had been ironed out and a sense of belief had been firmly instilled in the country.

India was on track to protect not just the vulnerable population but all citizens against a possible third wave of the disease. People understood how the vaccines worked. The mortality rate, the severity of the disease as well as its spread had reduced in India and around the world as vaccination numbers increased. It was clear that vaccines were immensely useful in reducing the severity of the disease. A vaccinated individual could contract Covid-19 or, in fact, even contract it repeatedly. But the chances of the disease being a big threat were reduced.

This role of vaccines—reducing severity—was embraced by people at large. In the initial days of vaccine introduction, the commentary around the world was sketchy—some views touted vaccines as preventive or curative. These ideas evolved and the true role of the vaccines in the national strategy to combat Covid-19 was well established.

From the despair and uncertainty of the first half of 2021 to the hope, confidence and positivity of the second half of the year, the popular narrative had changed. Indian science, backed by the government, had managed to defy all odds. That the most ebullient manifestation of this achievement showed up on 17 September was a fitting tribute to the political leadership that ushered in this change.

12

2022: FROM STRENGTH TO STRENGTH

The Indian vaccination juggernaut had well and truly captured 2021, proving every person who was eyeing India with scepticism wrong. The country had bounced back very strongly from the low points of the pandemic. The GDP had grown 20.1 per cent in the first quarter of the financial year 2021–22, 8.4 per cent in the second quarter, 5.4 per cent in the third quarter and 4.1 per cent in the fourth quarter. This amounted to 8.7 per cent growth for the full financial year.[1]

The country had lost one financial year due to the pandemic, but, by the end of the next fiscal, India had not only regained the economic activity levels of the pre-pandemic period, the growth trajectory had also almost normalized.

But the pandemic itself was not over. As several parts of the world were witnessing relative calm in the last quarter of 2021, a new variant of Covid-19 broke the creeping complacency. In November, South Africa and Botswana reported a new variant that was not only growing very fast but seemed to reinfect individuals who had previously suffered from the virus. This variant also seemed to be bypassing the immune protection offered by the vaccines. On 26 November, the WHO designated the strain, known as B.1.1.529, as a variant of concern and named it Omicron.[2]

This variant was considered so powerful in its mutations and potential ill-effects that several countries that had started to relax their Covid-19 measures immediately reversed the relaxations.

New curbs were quickly imposed, international conferences cancelled and borders closed. It was not clear what the real impact of this variant would be. However, given its significant potency, the Omicron variant immediately got treated with the same level of concern and escalation as the virus had been first subjected to in March 2020.

Ironically, Botswana and South Africa, which had acted with great responsibility in warning the world about a potential new problem, themselves got subjected to the harshest control measures. Many countries acted to stop travel and contact with the countries in the southern part of Africa as a response to this notification. They were penalized for guiding the world, demonstrating how the pandemic was not just attributable to biology but there was another parallel pandemic of lopsided perceptions and narratives going on. In fact, these countries had grappled with the conundrum whether they should talk about the new variant and do the right thing.[3]

It later turned out that the Omicron variant was already present in Europe.[4] The African nations just brought out its presence and worked on the sequencing of this variant. However, it was perhaps too late for the world as a whole to act specifically on this variant. In the US, the seven-day average death toll, after hitting a low of 797 on 27 November, started to rise through December. This average climbed to 1,328 deaths on 1 January and peaked at 2,670 deaths on 7 February.[5]

While the western world was in the grip of a new frenzy, India had a much better start to 2022. India did see a third wave of the pandemic, which began early January and peaked on 24 January 2022, but, by the end of February, the national daily case count was again back to very small numbers. The death toll ticked up a bit, but it was nowhere close to what the countries like the US or those in Europe had witnessed through their Omicron wave.

In quantitative terms, India saw more peak active daily cases during the Omicron wave (1.55 lakh on 11 January 2022) than during the Delta wave (1.35 lakh).[6] Crucially, however, India also saw a far higher recovery rate during the Omicron wave. Mortality numbers stayed above 1,000 every day between early April and late June during the Delta wave. The Omicron wave was very different—daily mortality in excess of 1,000 was seen for a short period between end of January and second week of February, peaking at around 1,700 versus more than 4,500 during the Delta wave.

In terms of raw numbers, 160 crore or 1.6 billion vaccines had been administered when the Omicron wave hit. Over 70 crore or 700 million people had been fully vaccinated with two doses, most of them within the previous six months. Keeping in mind that less than 40 per cent of the population of India lives in urban space, the cities were almost completely saturated in terms of vaccination coverage, and so were large parts of suburban and semi-rural areas. The consequences of the effort were clear—despite Omicron's ability to break through the vaccine defenses, the vaccination programme ensured only a brief uptick in mortality for two weeks and then dropped off, despite the active case count exceeding the Delta wave.

One study found that the impact of the Omicron variant in India was significantly milder due to the hybrid immunity Indians had developed.[7] The high degree of exposure to the virus during the Delta wave and a big part of the population getting vaccinated prevented a large-scale outbreak of infection.

Gavi made a similar observation: 'The good news is that the combination of vaccinations and natural immunity means many Indians are likely to have some degree of T cell immunity to SARS-CoV-2.'[8]

While the Delta wave was quite severe worldwide and there was no realistic chance of any country preventing the losses incurred in that wave, India's vaccination ramp-up through the year in 2021 certainly seemed to have a salubrious impact on the Omicron wave. Even later in the year, there were no large-scale outbreaks going into the summer of 2022, which had not been kind at all in the two previous years.

Vaccination Expands

While different parts of the world struggled in different measures through the first half of 2022, the focus in India was to recalibrate and expand the vaccination programme.

PM Modi addressed the nation on 25 December 2021 to make two key announcements. Firstly, India expanded the vaccination drive to youngsters. Those aged between 15 and 18 were now eligible for vaccination. This segment was allowed to be administered Covaxin, bringing in about 7.5 crore new estimated individuals in the vaccination net.

Secondly, India also started allowing a precaution dose for the healthcare and frontline workers, citizens who were over 60 years of age and those who had comorbidities. Many countries had started the process of booster vaccination doses and, in fact, had made it mandatory as part of vaccine passports being used in various social settings.

India's precaution dose approach was, again, well-timed with the rise of the Omicron wave, focussed on protecting those likely to be impacted most by a fresh outbreak. India also named the third dose as 'precaution' rather than a booster. This subtle difference also demonstrated how the Indian approach to the vaccination programme factored in all stakeholders.

The term 'booster' could easily morph into its plural form 'boosters'. In fact, Israel was one of the earliest countries to start administering a fourth dose of the vaccine to the vulnerable segments of the population. Later, a study[9] demonstrated that even a fourth dose was not good enough to protect the recipient against the infection itself, although, of course, the severity of the infection reduced.

Theoretically speaking, it may be possible for an individual to keep getting booster shots against the virus at periodic intervals, just like flu vaccines are administered in the western countries every year. But what would be the impact of multiple doses of Covid-19 vaccines on individuals? What would be the right gap between two booster doses? Would the benefit of multiple boosters outweigh the cost of the subsequent outbreaks of the pandemic, which was likely to become endemic over time?[10]

The balance of evidence was not strong enough to suggest that an endless series of booster doses may either be required or help if administered. Interestingly, PM Modi chose to use the term 'precaution' and not 'booster', when the third dose of the vaccine was made available.

The term very clearly suggested that it would be most relevant for those vulnerable and this relevance could be graded if the risks of a new variant or a new outbreak increased. One would take precaution in the wake of a risk perception, not just as a matter of an annual ritual. This subtle differentiation between booster and precaution also made it clear that the government was not expecting a run on the existing vaccine stocks. The intent was to target only those who required a third dose, and not restart a full universal vaccination programme again.

Following the announcement on 25 December, Mandaviya reviewed[11] India's preparedness for any potential Omicron wave and the status of the vaccination process with the health ministers of states on 2 January 2022. He praised the states' efforts in boosting vaccination drives and emphasized the importance of collective action. Through the acrimony and bitterness of 2021, India's vaccination scale-up had created a positive shift in the domestic perceptions of how the country dealt with the virus. Mandaviya's review, along with the PM regularly engaging with CMs, further helped in creating a favourable atmosphere for interstate cooperation.

This was a key message just before the vaccination began for those aged between 15 and 18.

Young India Believes

The registrations for the age group of 15–18 on CoWIN commenced on the first day of the new year. On the very first day of the vaccination, on 3 January, more than 40 lakh or 4 million doses were administered.[12] The total population in the said age group was estimated to be 7.5 crore or 75 million. The first day's response showed how eager young India was to bolster its bodily defenses against the virus.

World over, the young had been the least impacted by the virus. The number of cases, severe infections, hospitalizations as well as deaths were all significantly lower for those under 25 years of age, in comparison to the other age cohorts. There was, hence, an apprehension that the young population in India may want to skip vaccination.

Another viewpoint was that unlike the adults, there was only one vaccine available for those in the age group of 15–18. The lack of choice could have stopped many of them may from coming forward for vaccination. These theories were partly a continuation of the Made in India Covaxin scepticism, where the efforts to run down the legitimacy of the vaccine had never ended, despite its strong performance. However, young India trusted Covaxin as well as the vaccination process itself.

In 2020, the pandemic-led shutdown had come at the heels of the high school examinations and had led to higher secondary school examinations being wrapped up in a hurry. As these exams got over in March, India had gone ahead with a lockdown. This generation was the worst-impacted in terms of learning and self-development. These youngsters missed two critical and formative years of academic and social interactions, which help shape one's life ahead. Many college-goers did not see their college until late in the second year. Many who completed Class X were forced into remote learning or being home-schooled for the two remaining years of their school life.

Some in the 15–18 age group were victims of losing out on the opportunities to develop social skills. Others observed their siblings, friends and neighbours going through a tough mental adjustment of undertaking critical years of education without the requisite human touch.

Perhaps, it was factors like these that amplified the yearning for normalcy. Perhaps it was the recognition that a fresh Omicron outbreak may coincide with the higher secondary school examinations in 2022 and a repeat of the last two years would have been grossly devastating.

Whatever be the motivation, the late teens in India embraced science as staunchly and confidently as the adults had. Eventually, this group was administered over 6 crore or 60 million first doses. Schools and colleges worked normally through 2022, barring some localized instances of shutdowns lasting a few days due to an increase in the case count.

The Made in India Covaxin protected the next generation Indians in a critical phase of their life.

One-Year Anniversary

India marked a year of vaccinating its people on 15 January 2022. If on this day a year earlier—the day before the first vaccine dose was administered—someone would have predicted that India would finish with 156.02 crore or 1.56 billion vaccine doses a year later, such a guess would have been immediately dismissed as a flight of fancy.

But at the turn of Makar Sankranti, the festival that marks new beginnings, new harvests and longer days, symbolized by the flight of colourful kites adorning Indian skies, the number was real. The world's largest vaccination drive, with the potential exception of China, had well and truly delivered against all odds.

From the highest number of Day 1 vaccination across any country to the highest number of single-day vaccinations on

17 September 2021, India's vaccination drive had achieved several milestones en route.[13]

PM Modi summarized this one year aptly in a series of tweets on 16 January. He said: 'Today we mark #1YearOfVaccineDrive. I salute each and every individual who is associated with the vaccination drive. Our vaccination programme has added great strength to the fight against COVID-19. It has led to saving lives and thus protecting livelihoods.'[14]

'When the COVID-19 pandemic first struck, we did not know much about the virus. However, our scientists and innovators immersed themselves in developing vaccines. India feels proud that our nation has been able to contribute to fighting the pandemic through vaccines.'[15]

'At the same time, the role of our doctors, nurses and healthcare workers is exceptional. When we see glimpses of people being vaccinated in remote areas, or our healthcare workers taking the vaccines there, our hearts and minds are filled with pride.'[16]

'India's approach to fighting the pandemic will always remain science based. We are also augmenting health infrastructure to ensure our fellow citizens get proper care. Let us keep following all COVID-19 related protocols and overcome the pandemic. #1YearOfVaccineDrive.'[17]

PM Modi especially heralded the contribution of India's medical fraternity, which had tirelessly worked on treating as well as preventing the spread of the Covid-19 pandemic, oftentimes at great personal costs. He also stressed again that India's approach had been pro-science and guided by rational, data-driven policymaking.

Vaccine Arsenal Expands

On 22 February 2022, the DCGI gave emergency use approval for Corbevax to be administered to children.[18] The Hyderabad-based Biological E had been conducting trials for Corbevax, manufactured on the basis of the research conducted by the Baylor College of Medicine in Texas. This paved the path for immunization of children under 15 years of age.

Biological E had worked hard on this vaccine, collaborating with the team of Dr Peter Hotez, professor for paediatrics molecular virology at the Baylor College of Medicine and the researcher behind this vaccine. Dr Hotez had devised Corbevax as an ode to true decoloniality of vaccines[19], focussing on the ability of the developing countries to take the vaccine formulation and manufacture it themselves.

Dr Hotez worked backwards—his research took into account scalability and ease of production without the considerations of intellectual property. This is how his team focussed on the receptor binding domain, protein subunit vaccine, a platform that would be easily understood and scaled around the world.[20] However, transferring the technology for vaccines when the world was in the middle of shutdowns was not easy. The entire transfer of technology happened on video calls, with the Baylor College team helping the scientists from Biological E in assays. The scientists and chemists in India were able to use the initial set of vaccines and constituents shipped from the US and the knowledge of molecular biology imparted over video calls to reproduce the vaccine in India and then increase its production.[21]

A few weeks later in April,[22] Covaxin was granted EUA for children in the age group of 6–12, Corbevax for children in the age group 5–12 and ZyCoV-D to be used for children in the age group 12–18.

These approvals completed India's vaccine arsenal across all age groups and provided the flexibility to use different vaccines for different age groups based on clinical effectiveness, safety results and availability.

Criticism Continues

There are several ways to work towards an end goal and different individuals may evaluate the efficacy of different paths differently. Therefore, it is no surprise that the Indian vaccination programme also continued to attract critics late into 2021. Towards the end of the year, however, the criticism was blunted by the superlative performance of the vaccination drive.

The potential onset of the Omicron wave breathed fresh life into the somnolent compulsive contrarians. A spate of articles masquerading as expert analysis hit international media, announcing the oncoming period of difficulty for India. The theme was a repetitive one—India has not done enough and learnt no lessons from the past and, hence, it faces a disaster in the form of the Omicron variant.

The New York Times, which remained at the forefront of finding faults in India's Covid-19 response and inventing them when it could not find any, published an article titled 'India's Rising Omicron Wave Brings a Grim Sense of Déjà Vu' and subtitled it 'Just months after delta fuelled hospital failures and funeral pyres, India's leaders again offer a mixed message.'[23]

The Economist asked almost gleefully, 'Is India Prepared for Omicron?' It then pompously declared in the subtitle: 'Some lessons have been learnt from the devastating delta wave of 2021, but not all.'[24]

Unfortunately for those wiping the dust off their camera lenses, readying themselves to practise vulture journalism in India's graveyards, seeking to capture funeral pyres, none of this grim prognosis came true.

Although Omicron did lead to high case count in January and February 2022, its impact was a whimper. The government's own estimates for the case count were quite high. IISc, Bengaluru, and the Indian Statistical Institute, Kolkata, had predicted a million cases a day by the end of January.[25] The Susceptible,

Undetected, Tested (positive), and Removed, Analysis or SUTRA model developed by the Indian Institute of Technology, Kanpur, forecast 1.8 lakh cases by the first week of March at the peak of the Omicron wave.[26] This number was revised upwards in a later analysis.

On 22 January, India saw more than 3.33 lakh Covid-19 cases, after which the Omicron wave receded as quickly as it had climbed. The vaccines had presumably worked, certainly in terms of reducing the impact of the virus and perhaps in reducing the transmissibility.

Those who were waiting for a new wave of economic and social catastrophe in India were disappointed. This situation is best captured by a statement made by author Manu Joseph in an unrelated context, but fitting how Covid-19 analysis progressed in India: 'When the analysis of an intellectual aligns perfectly with his hope, then it is usually hope and not analysis.'[27]

The Elephant Marches On

India observes National Vaccination Day, also known as the National Immunization Day, every year on 16 March. This day was first observed in 1995, when India started the pulse polio campaign to further awareness about the importance and benefits of vaccination. The original intent was to create this awareness for vaccinating newborns.

In 2022, the symbolism of this day was used to extend the Covid-19 immunization programme to children in the age group of 12–14. Health Minister Mansukh Mandaviya announced this on his Twitter feed on 14 March.[28] The government planned to use Corbevax for this age group, and it had already placed an advance order of 30 crore or 300 million doses.[29]

Just like the older children in the 15–18 age group, those in the 12–14 age group also took to the vaccination programme enthusiastically. With an estimated population cohort of 6.4 crore or 64 million, more than 4.5 crore or 45 million vaccine doses were administered in just two months.[30]

Unlike in the age group of 15–18, where the personal agency of the child would be significant, it was the parents who were the decision-makers for the children in the 12–14 age group. With a significantly low risk perception as well, there was no surprise that this group had a slower administration of vaccine relative to other age groups, despite impressive total numbers.

On 17 July 2022, India completed 2 billion vaccine doses. The milestone came within a year-and-a-half of the starting of the vaccinations. At this time, 90 per cent of adults were fully vaccinated and another 5 per cent had taken the first dose. About 50 per cent of the children between 12 and 18 years of age were also fully vaccinated.[31]

For a developing country running a vaccination programme purely with Made in India vaccines and hosting more than 17 per cent of the total world population, this was a stupendous effort. To top this, India also exported more than 27.16 crore or 271.6 million vaccine doses, helping fully vaccinate a substantial portion of the population of several countries.[32]

In less than 18 months, India had shielded itself and helped many around the world to do the same. Time is the best judge of success and undoubtedly, time indeed endorsed India's tenacity. Rabindranath Tagore once remarked: 'Facts are many, but the truth is one.' The only truth in the fight against Covid-19 was that the Indian vaccination story was an overwhelming success.

13

AN ACHIEVEMENT TO BE TRULY PROUD OF

India is classified as a lower middle-income developing country today, but it has always been a fertile and productive land. This has been historically proven. For approximately 2,000 years, the Indian subcontinent traded places with the Chinese eastern seaboard as the home to the largest concentration of people on Earth.

In the year 1000 CE, the most populous geographical entity was China, ruled by Song dynasty. The population of the regions that make up the modern nation state of India was amongst the highest in the world relative to other regions.[1] Other Indian dynasties also ranked on the list. Understood differently, India collectively was perhaps the most populous geographical entity 1,000 years ago. Some of the others were geographically larger, but only two had the ability to sustain a high population density for thousands of years—India and China.

Before industrialization, genetically enhanced crop yields and modern medicine, life on Earth was unforgiving. When the tipping point of the ability of land to sustain a population was crossed, the result was tragic, typically in the form of famines. If there were too many mouths to feed, people died or dispersed and tried to rebuild life elsewhere. This was the harsh manner in which nature enforced the balance between resources and population. In short, it was simply not possible to artificially maintain a large population for a long period—nature would brutally correct the imbalance.

The Indian subcontinent could not have sustained a population exceeding all of Europe for thousands of years without being a fertile and productive place for human life to prosper. That's not to suggest there were no famines in Indian history. There were several—particularly the ones during the British rule, when a combination of high farm taxation and export ravaged the Indian economy—and yet, India remained a very densely populated region for essentially all of recorded history.

Slices of India Population vs Whole Countries

Table 11 shows how narrow population cohorts in India can be bigger than entire countries. Each Indian demographic cohort is enumerated and their size compared to a reasonably large country for a contextual purpose.

TABLE 11

Appreciating Indian Population Scale[2]

Population Group (age)	*Approximate size (in million)*	*Comparable Countries*
0–4	115	UK + Spain
5–9	117	France + Spain
10–14	125	Japan
15–19	125	Japan
20–24	122	Japan
25–29	120	France + Italy
30–34	112	Italy + South Korea
35–39	105	UK + Canada
40–44	90	Spain + Ukraine
45–49	80	Germany
50–54	70	South Korea + Netherlands
55–59	60	South Africa
60+	125	Japan

Therefore, when India announced vaccination for the age groups of 12–14 and 15–17—each approximately 80 million strong—it amounted to an institutional preparedness to vaccinate the equivalent of Germany's population in short order.

India administered first doses to approximately 70 per cent of the 15–17 age group in a month and a half.[3] Germany, a vastly developed and modern country and the home of BioNTech, Bayer, Hoechst, CureVac, among others, did so in 11 months.[4]

Numbers themselves are not sufficient for anyone to contextualize the scale of the challenge. A simple recent argument like 'the government must offer boosters to everyone in the 45–59 age group' translates to the need to organize and carry out 210 million additional vaccinations, exceeding the population of Japan and Germany combined.

Also consider the timeframe—these countries took close to a year to administer vaccinations amongst 70 per cent of their populations as far as first dose coverage was concerned. Let's say the goal is to administer booster dose among the 45–59 age group within a span of three months. That amounts to a request to not only execute the equivalent of the programmes in those two countries *combined* but also *four times faster*. Not just that, the challenge also involves being able to do so on top of all the other ongoing medical requirements and other vaccination activities.

This isn't to argue that the problem is so hard that it can't be solved. It *already* was in several ways. In December 2021, 211 million vaccinations were performed. In January 2022, the number was 215 million. In September 2021, which was the zenith, India administered nearly 240 million vaccinations[5]—the equivalent of the combined total population of France, Italy, Spain and UK being inoculated once. These are just one month numbers—the comparable countries individually took around a year to carry out the same number of vaccinations.

Multiple population cohorts received vaccination doses at a rate up to an order of magnitude (10 times) faster than the corresponding country equivalent. Between June 2021 and February 2022, there were nine consecutive months when more than 100 million doses were administered. From August to January 2021, each month exceeded 170 million doses. Three of those exceeded 200 million doses each month.

Even looking at major transnational agglomerations, such as North America or the EU, India's demographic weight is far bigger. Both these entities, for example, have a smaller population than even northern India. The whole of Europe has a population approximately that of northern and western Indian states combined.

The Indian vaccination programme has been carried out with little divergence in vaccination rates across states—geographical accessibility is the most common impediment in comparison to any political boundary. As of June 2022, India vaccinated a larger share of its total population—73 per cent,[6] which was greater than North America (72 per cent) or Europe (69 per cent).[7]

This is despite the sum of their populations adding up to India's total population and the fact that India has a far younger population and thus a much larger share of population that cannot yet be vaccinated. India approved vaccination for those aged between 12 and 18 years of age in phases in 2022. Despite starting with a lag for every cohort, India's vaccination rates continued to be higher than those in North America or Europe.

Nudging Public Demand Behaviour

Through the course of the vaccination process, the government had to constantly consider a key question: who should be eligible to receive the vaccine? Given that all countries, including India, applied, the implicit idea was that some manner of grouping was necessary to ensure effective execution. The alternative, of course, was to open up vaccination eligibility to entire swathes of the population. But this would have only led to further vaccine hesitancy.

The term 'vaccine hesitancy' is often poorly articulated or outright misused. The more trivial explanation is the literal one—people aren't getting vaccinated. It makes no effort to explain the broadly identifiable individual reasoning, general causative bases or any external factors affecting the visible end result.

If vaccinations were opened up to a much larger cohort than the available vaccine production rate, it would have led to packed vaccination centres, people repeatedly looking for reservations on CoWIN and that would have ultimately led to crashing of the website. This would have made Covid-19 vaccination yet another victim of India's perennial public goods supply shortages that have been witnessed over the decades and are still found in pockets like urban transportation. People would have thronged vaccination centres only to be turned back. They would have perhaps tried one or two more times at the most, and then would have decided that there was a 'vaccine shortage'. And they would have been right in saying so—from their point of view, there would be a shortage regardless of whether 1 million or 10 million vaccinations were being performed per day till the time they were vaccinated.

Negative experiences of this kind could have resulted in wide-ranging breakdown in the entire vaccination effort. The story of 'vaccine shortage' would have resulted in a broadly passive disengagement from the vaccination effort and consequent vaccine hesitancy.

Willing people returning unvaccinated would have led to distrust in the execution process. Those giving up due to this distrust would have continued to be at risk of being impacted more harshly by Covid-19. This would have led to a larger problem of greater rate of transmission, which would have further pressured the healthcare systems.

The pithy conclusion that many in the commentariat reached to avoid such possibilities was 'produce more'. This gross oversimplification sounded good on social media or on television shows, but was divorced from reality—production and consumption are dynamic parameters that need constant rate management.

As a corollary, the vaccination effort demonstrated that people were willing to wait for their turn and step forward when their eligibility was announced. An implicit social contract between the public and the government was witnessed here. As much as the people were anxious to be vaccinated, they did fundamentally recognize and agree with the prioritization process.

The public recognized that the aged, frail and immunocompromised were at maximum risk and, hence, needed to be prioritized. They recognized that it is a saner approach to create eligibility groups in descending order from the most vulnerable to the least. They recognized that there is no point in giving false hope about vaccine availability—it would be a waste of their time and would harm the credibility of their overall effort.

This nuanced understanding of the right way to execute such an effort was one of the several ways in which the government understood the critical importance of effective execution from the macro to micro levels. It wasn't simply enough to have good intentions—the population would not have benefitted if execution on the ground was poor.

Two major factors define the vaccination organization. First is the medical basis behind the creation of groups, driven by the relative risk factors that are broadly related to a person's age, and second is the logistical factor that aligns supply with demand in a manner that it matches the rates. Both the factors will be described in more detail.

Understanding Vaccination Strategy

Two documents were published by the Ministry of Health and Family Welfare and the ICMR in the autumn and early winter of 2020, respectively: the Covid-19 Vaccine Operational Guidelines[8] and Covid-19 Vaccine Communications Strategy.[9]

The documents addressed everything from defining priority groups, to details on effective communication strategies, mitigating vaccine hesitancy, tracking of AEFI i.e., vaccine side effects, and more.

The topic of prioritization groups was covered in the Covid-19 Vaccine Operational Guidelines:

- Health Care Workers (HCWs): The actual health professionals who organize and perform the vaccination
- Frontline Workers (FLWs): The support personnel who help organize the vaccination operations—municipal and civil service personnel, the armed forces and police members all deputed to the task
- Prioritized age groups, starting with those over 60 years of age, then the 50–59 year-old group (later amended to the 45–59 year-old group) and then the 18–44 year-old group, and finally the youth and children's groups.[10]

With some variation, every major country did the same thing. Some combined the vaccination of HCWs and FLWs with the vaccination of the highest risk groups. This was also riskier as healthcare workers could infect the critically at-risk older patients in care centres.

The US started vaccinating HCWs and the highest risk groups at the same time, but this was because of western culture enabling the old to be placed in care centres, which were epicentres of high mortality in the US—by autumn of 2020, more than 1,700 American healthcare workers had died[11] of Covid-19. As of February 2022, over 2 lakh healthcare workers and support staff died[12] of Covid-19 in the US.

The US and western Europe, therefore, did not have much choice. Given the relatively high mortality rates predating vaccinations despite their best efforts to prevent transmission of the virus from hospital personnel to patients, they were forced to start early.

India's situation was more fraught. With far greater population densities and fewer healthcare workers per 1,000 people, this would mean far greater potential for the virus to be passed to several people by an asymptomatic healthcare worker during the actual process of vaccination. Therefore, the Indian policy—also used by Japan and several other nations—sought to first vaccinate HCWs and FLWs, and then the highest risk groups.

It has often been argued that the Indian vaccination efforts have been 'unscientific'. However, Indian prioritization efforts aligned with the most authoritative early investigations into Covid-19 mortality. Joshua R. Goldstein and Ronald D. Lee[13] reported as far back as August 2020 how Covid-related age-specific death rates (ASDRs) increased exponentially past the 60+ and especially 70+ age groups across several western nations.

Another notable accomplishment of this Covid-19 Vaccine Operational Guidelines document was that it described the architecture of the Covid-19 Vaccine Intelligence Network, popularly known as CoWIN. A perusal of the document demonstrates the early emphasis on this digital platform as a holistic solution to the logistical problem of vaccinating 1.37 billion people.

Not only did CoWIN enable registration on the consumer side, it enabled administrative planning and resource allocation behind the scenes. Vaccine registration data enabled decision-making on how to allocate and manage vaccinations down to individual primary and secondary healthcare centres, so that they could minimize wastage of vials that must be utilized within a certain number of hours after being opened.

Section 5.3 of the Covid-19 Vaccine Operational Guidelines document described training and organization of personnel at each vaccination centre, describing the division of roles and workflows.

It is important to emphasize that all these were defined in a document released in late 2020, well before the first dose of

Covid-19 vaccine was administered. In the 18 months since the release of the document, 2 billion doses of vaccines have been administered, and this system has been executed exactly as the operational document proposed.

Critical reviews have often taken self-congratulatory tones, suggesting the vaccination drive only became organized after being faced with strident criticism. In reality, the vaccination drive was executed almost exactly the way the original operational guidelines document prescribed, months before the first vaccine dose was administered.

Communication Planning

The Covid-19 Vaccine Communications Strategy document spends a significant amount of time on describing a bottom-up approach for communicating to the public the importance of the efforts being put into the eradication of Covid-19. The nuance of this approach deserves its own detailed overview.

Fundamentally, the communication strategy focussed far more upon last mile communication than it did on the top-down communication aspect. For example, the document described an information dissemination approach utilizing essentially every low-level grouping known—mahila mandals, self-help groups, panchayat leaders, resident welfare associations, Nehru Yuva Kendra Sangathan, National Service Scheme, swacchagrahis, nigrani samitis, mahila arogya samitis, gram sabhas, faith-based groups and more. Many states in India relied on communicating in local languages, which proved to be of immense help in making the vaccination appeal sharper and more relatable.[14]

This was dramatically different from the approach seen in most western nations, where the communication strategy was very top-down. Their approaches treated communication as a way to convey 'this is good for you and you should go get vaccinated because we're saying so from a position of authority and scientific basis'. Almost all American vaccine communication was associated with the nodal federal agency CDC or personalities like Dr Anthony Fauci, the chief medical advisor to the president of the US.

This would have been an extremely bad approach for mass vaccination in a large, diverse nation such as India. People would naturally have had a range of legitimate concerns about vaccines. People would have wished to have some trusted entity with whom they could have a conversation about their concerns regarding being vaccinated. The Indian approach focussed from the outset on a diffused delivery of the message through the vast array of low-level social organizations people affiliate with in some manner or the other.

The result of this approach can be seen in the manner in which the entire vaccination effort panned out. It would have been easy to envision entire swathes of the population refusing to be vaccinated because of their beliefs unrelated to science. This was quite literally the case in the US, where approximately 15 per cent of the population simply refused to get vaccinated because of various reasons—personal beliefs, social conditioning or political views.[15]

This nuanced approach to diffused communication was another example of the intelligence with which the government organized and executed the vaccination process. This reflected a deep understanding of both sociocultural concerns as well as the internalized experience from past efforts. A heavy-handed and authoritarian 'go get vaccinated if you know what's good for you' approach would have played into potential political fault lines that would have damaged the credibility of the vaccination effort.

The active dynamic of the local PHCs and CHCs was deliberately leveraged by the government. These centres served both as medical centres and a source of public healthcare reference and knowledge. These centres served as an effective mechanism to educate the public about the necessity of vaccination.[16] They enabled the dissemination of correct advice to the public.

This was the right approach to initiate interaction between the common man and public health officials—the most credible source of healthcare information is the healthcare system itself. Elsewhere—in the US, for example—the pandemic saw a breakdown in the trust between the public and the government to an alarming extent, with a section of the public choosing to get healthcare advice from a collection of dubious websites, demagogues and outright quacks.

The lack of a cohesive relationship between the public and their local healthcare system demonstrably made vaccination harder in many places, ranging from low-income countries with an under-developed healthcare system to developed countries where for-profit healthcare is unaffordable or inequitable.

This is particularly important to understand because such breakdowns occured in otherwise advanced and educated western countries, where one would not expect to normally see such behaviour.

India is a developing society with significantly lower levels of attainment in terms of education and access to knowledge of best healthcare practices. However, our existing infrastructure was used extremely effectively. The same public health system that educates women on effective birth control, prenatal, antenatal and paediatric care and offers broad public healthcare services came to the fore to drive the process of engaging the public on the importance of vaccination and proper pandemic health protocols.

India has, thus, seen essentially none of the almost bizarre levels of conspiracy theorizing and 'anti-vaxxer' movements as seen in the US and elsewhere. With resources for the general public to turn to in order to get their concerns and questions answered, the Indian process was remarkably smooth, with sustained high vaccination rates in every state, regardless of the political hues of the respective state administrations.

A Spirit of Trust and Collaboration

Through the vaccination effort, India demonstrated a very high level of organizational ability to execute a task at a scale where we have only one other peer of comparable size—China. While China administered far more vaccinations, they focussed on high-volume production of quickly approved vaccines, combined with an arguably overzealous 'Zero Covid' strategy. The efficacy of the vaccines has been in question on the basis of China's stringent curbs extending well into 2022. In effect, their approach may have been to give multiple booster doses and cover large parts of the population faster, rather than focussing on greater vaccine efficacy.

In comparison, India has largely been able to handle the pandemic. As of the end of June 2022, nearly 1.1 billion people in India were administered at least a single vaccine dose, and among them, 910 million received two doses and close to 50 million received three.[17]

The credit for these impressive statistics should go to a broadly cohesive interaction between the State and its people. The most sustainable story of the vaccination effort—which took off during the worst days of the second wave caused by the Delta variant—is that the public still fundamentally trusts an effective government.

Except for about six weeks in the middle of the Delta wave in April and May 2021, India's machinery largely seemed in control of the proceedings. The Delta wave was far too ferocious for the healthcare system, but even then, no efforts were spared to reverse the tide. In fact, the vaccination process continued to chug along, even when the infections led to large-scale disruptions in these six weeks.

India responded with a level of sophistication and maturity that belies the manner in which it is classified in the international political economy—as a lower-middle-income developing country. Implicit in this categorization is that the country has not developed the necessary state institutions and capacity to demonstrate state power that enables it to be categorized as a major developed power. During the course of 2021, the Indian public and State collaborated in a manner that underscores the sophistication of the social contract between the state and the citizenry. Rather than responding emotionally and—figuratively—going after the government with pitchforks and flaming torches, Indians were partners in the success.

What India demonstrated during the Covid-19 response is that we have a sophisticated public that understands the challenges of execution. It also recognizes both basic and sophisticated solutions being delivered to solve long-pending problems. People demonstrated that they understood that implementation of infrastructure is just one part of the solution. Their ability to observe and understand the execution of the solution forms another part of the solution.

This is best explained by looking at one's personal usage of CoWIN or the Aarogya Setu app. As early as March 2021, the app itself was available, even if the vaccine production was just ramping up. Everyone could see the vaccine registration and performance numbers. They may have tried and failed—potentially multiple times—to register themselves. But CoWIN treated people as part of the solution. It treated them as adults, helping them see what was happening. While their own turn to be vaccinated may not have come, there was observable movement and ability to understand how the process was evolving.

This matters enormously in ensuring the cohesion of the social contract between the State and its subjects. CoWIN or Aarogya Setu were not merely websites and apps but represented the State, informing the public in great detail, even in the midst of its most challenging period of vaccinations, that it was working hard. Such a mature and sophisticated interaction with the public received a mature response. People waited for their turn patiently and got vaccinated when they were eligible. All of this was done with no arbitrariness or graft. There was no hoarding and reselling of vaccines and hardly any VIP culture to complain about.

The government's Jan Dhan-Aadhaar-Mobile (JAM) project paid rich dividends, enabling the public to register for vaccinations and receive them in a technically sophisticated and seamless manner, nationwide.

Punching Above the Weight

It's tempting to be dismissive of this as 'oh, all the western nations have all this too'. However, they don't necessarily have such a system as CoWIN. The US, for example, does not have any national-level vaccine registration or tracking mechanism. Several American states have their own systems. In the case of those that do not, one calls around various places hoping to find a location that has an appointment available.

Developed countries are not merely characterized by their per capita income levels. While it may be true that India is far from a high-income nation, India's response to Covid-19 demonstrates that the country is among the best in the world at deploying its own local scientific, technical, manufacturing and organizational capabilities to independently perform at par with or better than every other highly populated nation or supranational entity in response to a pandemic-scale global emergency.

If we set the bar at geographical entities with populations exceeding 400 million, the comparison set would be China, India, Europe and North America. All four entities demonstrated the ability to develop and produce Covid-19 vaccines themselves at the necessary scale to vaccinate their individual populations—580 million for North America, 750 million for Europe, and 1.4 billion in the case of both China and India.[18]

If we set the bar lower, at 100 million as the baseline population, it would account for the top 12 most populous countries in the world. The top two—China and India—were self-sufficient in local production of the vaccine. In the third position, the US was partially self-sufficient, having received significant volumes of vaccines from American multinational production facilities in Europe.

The next several countries—Indonesia, Pakistan, Nigeria, Brazil and Bangladesh—all depended almost entirely on imported vaccines, with Brazil having some manufacturing capabilities. Next, Russia was self-sufficient but with only one option—the Sputnik V vaccine. Next was Mexico and Japan, both with limited local production capability and depending significantly on imports. The remaining members of the greater-than-100-million population club—Ethiopia, Philippines and Egypt—all depended on imports.

In effect, the pandemic has shown that the vast majority of the global vaccine production comes from three entities—China, India and the multinational pharmaceutical empires spread across the US and Europe.

Table 12 summarizes the true strength of India's vaccine manufacturing capacity. Vaccines that were authorized for imports have also been included for a complete picture of the Covid-19 vaccine universe in India.

Indian technology rose to the occasion, and not just for vaccine production.

TABLE 12

Covid-19 Vaccines Authorized for Use in India[19]

Vaccine Name	*Company Name*	*Manufacturing Unit Location*	*Approval Date by CDSCO (Restricted Use in Emergency)*	*Approved for Age Group*	*Date of Inclusion in National Vaccination Programme*	*Remarks*
Covishield	Serum Institute of India	Pune	3 January 2021	≥ 18 years	16 January 2021 for the age group of 18 years onwards	Market authorization given on 27 January 2022
Covaxin	Bharat Biotech	Hyderabad, Ankleshwar	3 January 2021	≥ 18 years	16 January 2021 for the age group of 18 years onwards	Market authorization given on 27 January 2022
			24 December 2021	≥ 12 to 18 years	3 January 2022 for the age group of 15–18 years	
			26 April 2022	> 6 to <12 years		

CorBEvax	Biological E Limited	Hyderabad	28 December 2021	≥ 18 years		
			21 February 2022	≥ 12 years	16 March 2022 for the age group of 12–14 years (both government and private centres) 5 May 2022 for the age group of 15–17 years (private centres only) 28 June 2022 for the age group of 18 years onwards (private centres only)	
			26 April 2022	≥ 5 to < 12 years		

Sputnik V	Dr. Reddy's Lab (Importer)	Hyderabad	12 April 2021	≥ 18 years	12 May 2021 for those older than or equal to 18 years of age (private centres only)	
	Panacea Biotec	New Delhi	2 July 2021	≥ 18 years		
	Hetero Biopharma	Hyderabad	7 October 2021	≥ 18 years		
Sputnik Light	Dr. Reddy's Lab (Importer)	Hyderabad	5 February 2022	≥ 18 years		
	Hetero Biopharma	Hyderabad	16 March 2022	≥ 18 years		
Zycov-D	Cadila Healthcare	Ahmedabad	20 August 2021	≥ 12 years	26 November 2021 for >18 years	Three doses; Day 0, 28, 56
			26 April 2022	≥ 12 years		Two doses; Day 0, 28

Covovax	Serum Institute of India	Pune	28 December 2021	≥ 18 years		
			8 March 2022	≥ 12 years	5 May 2022 for the age group of 15–17 years (private centres only) 28 June 2022 (centres only)	
Moderna	Cipla (Importer)	Mumbai	29 June 2021	≥ 18 years	Not introduced	
Janssen Vaccine	Johnson & Johnson (Importer)		7 August 2021	≥ 18 years	Not introduced	
	Biological E	Hyderabad	18 August 2021	≥ 18 years	Not introduced	

14

POWER OF PUBLIC DIGITAL INFRASTRUCTURE

Public digital infrastructure, also referred to as digital public goods, has become a popular term in the last few years. Governments using technology to deliver public services more productively is not a new concept. But the rapid evolution of data storage, processing and insight-generation capabilities have got governments around the world thinking about creating public digital infrastructure, which helps in not just efficient governance but a total reimagination of how governments can connect with their citizens.

'Government 2.0, then, is the use of technology—especially the collaborative technologies at the heart of Web 2.0—to better solve collective problems at a city, state, national, and international level,' Tim O'Reilly, CEO of O'Reilly Media said in a paper published in 2010.[1] This paper is considered the origination of the 'Government as a Platform', a concept that got popularized as public digital infrastructure as well as assets and goods, in subsequent technology writing.

India's push for public digital infrastructure started in August 2014. In his first speech from the ramparts of the Red Fort in New Delhi, PM Narendra Modi vowed[2] that digital infrastructure was critical to empower citizens. The first such infrastructure programme on financial inclusion, named Jan Dhan Yojana, was also launched in this speech.

As mobile phones permeated within society, India went from a connectivity-starved country to having the highest per capita data consumption and one of the lowest rates for per gigabyte of mobile data in the world. In parallel, the public service delivery was scaling through the use of Aadhaar, the 12-digit biometric identity assigned to every resident Indian. Eventually, the runaway success of this JAM trinity paved the way for a national embrace of the concept of public digital infrastructure.

Technology: Sine Qua Non

Through the various review meetings in 2020, PM Modi continued to emphasize that the vaccination programme had to be technology-enabled. On the supply side, the use of the eVIN was finalized through the second half of the year. Since this platform was already available for the existing immunization programmes, it was a natural choice for managing the supply and tracking of Covid-19 vaccines.

On 30 May 2020, PM Modi invited[3] Ram Sewak Sharma, then chairman of the Telecom Regulatory Authority of India, for a meeting. This meeting was to discuss using technology for the smooth running of the vaccination process in the country. At this stage, there were no vaccines and no plan for a national vaccination drive. But the government was cognizant of challenges that a nationwide vaccination drive would face in execution. There was also a keen belief that the use of technology could potentially help in this massive nationwide exercise.

Sharma, who had headed the Unique Identification Authority of India (UIDAI), the body that drove the issuance and adoption of Aadhaar, made a presentation to the PM. This presentation emphasized why an Aadhaar-linked record of vaccination was important to be maintained.

However, the question of a citizen-facing front-end platform remained open. The prevalent thought was that the eVIN could be repurposed as a front-end application, too. But the challenge of implementing such a system was non-trivial in nature. It was obvious that if a digital platform was to be used for bookings, confirmation and verification of vaccine doses, it would have to be hugely scalable, given the Indian population base.

This citizen-facing platform was to be called CoWIN. The government sought the help of India's vibrant technology sector and start-ups to scale-up the platform and make it ready for nationwide use.[4] This effort was over and above the work already being done within the government. These efforts did not fully result in a system that could support a nationwide programme.

Since the first set of vaccine recipients was a controlled set of healthcare workers and frontline workers, the health ministry believed that repurposing the eVIN could work. The target population in this cohort was about 3 crore. There was a growing realization that as the total number of potential vaccine recipients increased, the system requirements would also become onerous.

The repurposed version of the eVIN was peer-reviewed[5] on 24 December 2020 under the chairmanship of Dr V.K. Paul. The experts invited for this review included Nandan Nilekani, the original architect of Aadhaar and the non-executive chairman of Infosys, J. Satyanarayana, then-chairman of the UIDAI, Ajay Sawhney, then secretary of the Ministry of Electronics and Information Technology, Dr Neeta Verma, then director general of the National Informatics Centre, Abhishek Singh, the CEO of the National e-Governance Division, and Pramod Verma, chief architect of the UIDAI.

CoWIN was tested[6] on 28 and 29 December 2020 at five sites each in the states of Andhra Pradesh, Assam, Gujarat and Punjab for readiness and to get user feedback. Subsequently, on 4 January 2021, the platform was tested in 125 districts around the country with 286 mock vaccination sessions created and managed through the platform. On 8 January 2021, a week before the launch, CoWIN was tested in more than 700 districts around the country to ensure healthcare workers and public health officials were familiar with it.

Meanwhile, PM Modi continued to emphasize in his regular review meetings that the success of the digital platform was a must. India would not be adopting any paper-based process at any point of time, so the digital platform had to scale-up elegantly. The PM raised issues like the international recognition of certificates and emphasized that India had to be prepared in the best possible manner to ensure that proof of vaccination would not be questioned. He also wanted to ensure that the second dose tracking was done systematically, as the concerns regarding vaccine complacency as well as hesitancy were real.

Sensing that the technological backbone would need further robustness, PM Modi decided to revive the team that had delivered Aadhaar. On 7 January 2021, he called[7] Ram Sewak Sharma. The PM had a vivid recollection of the May 2020 conversation with Sharma. He stressed on the technology imperatives for a successful vaccination process and asked Sharma to join the team of experts, which was working on this endeavour.

Sharma, an Indian Administrative Service (IAS) officer of the Jharkhand cadre from 1978, had retired from government service at the end of September 2020. He was at his ancestral village near Firozabad in Uttar Pradesh, when he was recalled to join the management of the vaccination process.

Sharma was appointed the head of the Empowered Group on Technology and Data Management and was also appointed as a member of the NEGVAC administration. Then, at the end of January 2021, he took over as the CEO of the National Health Authority.

With the PM's intervention, the team that worked with Sharma at the UIDAI was brought back to shore up the technological backbone. On 14 January 2021, two days before India's vaccination drive started, Sharma met the PM with bad news. The platform was not fully functional yet. A lot of work was still required and he was expecting the PM to be unhappy with the assessment.

PM Modi, instead, instructed[8] Sharma to ensure that the digital platform was fully scaled by the time the second dose was administered to the healthcare and frontline workers. In effect, there was a month to ensure that the technology held up.

The vision that PM Modi put forward for the technology had four guiding principles.[9] First, technology had to ensure that the vaccination process was equitable and inclusive across multilingual states, where multiple modes for registration to ensure accessibility for all should be possible. Second, India needed a single source of truth that could be used for unbiased distribution of vaccine information through a single source of data to remove information asymmetry and align all stakeholders. Third, the application should have a dynamic architecture, capable of evolving and accommodating changes as per the circumstances, and built for a scale of a billion-plus citizens. Fourth, data on vaccination and recording of adverse events should help in the formulation of data-driven public health policy and help in evaluating the efficacy of different vaccines.

Sturdy Architecture

On 16 January 2021, India launched the vaccination programme on CoWIN. From day one, the entire process was digitized. Sharma's five-member team continued to work on the application. They took the fundamental view that no single website may be able to handle the volume of concurrent users accessing the system from around the country. Hence, they worked on creating a robust back-end platform while taking the approach of publishing application programming interfaces (APIs) to ensure that various front-end applications could connect to the platform for specific functions.

The robustness of the back-end became the primary consideration for Sharma's team. They put lessons from the Aadhaar platform development to good use. The CoWIN platform was developed with a classic three-layer architecture.[10]

The CoWIN portal, which the users used for viewing available slots and booking, formed the front end. The CoWIN dashboard, which was published for public viewing and near-real-time tracking of vaccination processes, was designed as the information front end.

The business functionality was contained in the middle layer of the architecture, which was itself divided in four modules—registration and scheduling, vaccination facility, vacation and certificate. Each of these four modules were connected with their respective databases, storing relevant data in the third layer of the architecture.

This technology architecture promoted the use of APIs.[11] Third-party applications could use these interfaces to interact with specific modules and help users undertake a task related to that module.

The registration and scheduling application programming interfaces enabled the development of applications that provided more front-end interfaces to let citizens register for vaccination. These applications also allowed the discovery of available vaccination slots and scheduling or rescheduling of appointments.

The vaccination facilities application programming interfaces allowed government and private hospitals to link their existing systems to CoWIN. These vaccination sites could also record vaccination data for certification. These sites were also facilitated with reporting of adverse events for any impacted beneficiary.

Finally, the certification application programming interfaces allowed portals like corporate building management systems or travel portals to access vaccination certificates based on a reference identification or a registered mobile number to validate vaccination status of individuals.

These functions of CoWIN were seen and used by all Indian citizens who opted for vaccination. The functionalities for the vaccinators and the public health officials of all districts also tied in seamlessly.

The vaccinators could manage the schedule of the sessions assigned to them. They could also verify the identification details of the citizens who showed up at their centres.

Like the users, hospitals were also on-boarded on the CoWIN platform, with designated public health officials getting the administrative rights for managing the district-level processes. These managers could create and update vaccination facility details, create and update details of vaccination sessions, see the details across districts and map vaccine availability in their districts.

CoWIN was going to get significantly more traffic than Aadhaar systems, given its in-built necessity of concurrency. Every platform usage experience had to be good, or else people would quickly lose trust in the technology.

This problem was further compounded by the fact that not all Indians would be able to use the technology with equal facility. Registrations and recording of data would require intervention by the technicians working on vaccination sites when people walked in to receive vaccination doses.

The system was designed to work with Aadhaar as the central reference number, as has been the case for all of India's public digital infrastructure. Every user could register with a mobile phone and Aadhaar reference, which would then record both doses against the mentioned Aadhaar number. Since Aadhaar use was not mandatory, the system also had the provision for users to register with other identity numbers. Nonetheless, unique identification of the user was a key feature of the system and the central tenet on which it was designed.

The International Contrast

While a lot of CoWIN features sounded perfectly logical, and, in hindsight, even simplistic, the importance of a technology-validated, no-manual-intervention system was not fully appreciated until late into the vaccination process. As is often the case, contrasting experience helps in appreciating the true value of what's commonplace.

By August 2021, there was a flourishing black market in the US for manual vaccination cards, which were being used throughout the country.[12] The state of New York was trying to bring vaccine forgeries to justice[13] as late as January 2022, more than 13 months after the US started the vaccination process. It was only in February 2022 when the US FDA warned that vaccine forgeries were a problem to be aware of.[14]

In April 2022, *The New York Times* reported that the Justice Department had charged 21 individuals for vaccine fraud, which also included selling fake vaccination proofs.[15] The same story also reported that 'in New Jersey, prosecutors charged a Postal Service employee with making and distributing 400 fake vaccination cards, in part to "undermine" the federal government's role in ensuring that people comply with public health requirements, according to prosecutors".'[16]

Despite these widespread irregularities, the international media, including *The New York Times*, did not allude to the American vaccination process being a failure. Of course, that would have been a very unjust and far-reaching allegation. But then, in contrast, the same media had been using India's episodic issues to project a narrative of national failures throughout the pandemic reporting.

Not just fake vaccine certificates, the US had an even bigger logistical issue when it came to tracking vaccinations. It was essentially left to the individuals to ensure that they had taken the stipulated two doses in the original vaccination process. Since an individual could take the two doses at two different locations, even across cities and states, not just different facilities, there was no central tracking system in place. If an individual was to use two different facilities, it was common for both the facilities to chase[17] the person concerned to 'take the second dose'.

And this was not just the US. Even smaller and significantly richer countries, like Switzerland, had problems. In December 2021, an enquiry was launched[18] when the local authorities discovered around 8,000 fake vaccination cards in the eastern canton of St. Gallen. One of the richest cantons—the Swiss equivalent of states—in a country that stands very high in global per capita income also could not prevent fake certificates. For reference, the cantonal population of St. Gallen's is estimated to be just over half a million. The 8,000 fake certificates equate to 1.5 per cent of the total cantonal population and an even higher percentage of the population eligible for vaccination.

In December 2021, France detected more than 180,000 fake Covid-19 passes, which also included fake certificates.[19] Around the same time, Italy made arrests for false inoculations.[20] In Austria, the local police uncovered widespread fake certificate fraud again in December 2021.[21]

These situations further elaborated the importance of CoWIN. Since the international recognition of vaccine certificates was integral for the post-pandemic world, India had to set a high bar, unfortunately higher than what other countries could get away with, of demonstrating a robust process.

Agile Adjustments and Problem Solving

This is not to say that CoWIN did not have problems. It was natural that a system of this scale and magnitude went through an initial phase of turbulence.

The first spike in the use of CoWIN came when India opened vaccination for all individuals who were 45 and above on 1 April. As the eligible base expanded, the CoWIN platform had to support an expanded set of registrations overnight. At this stage, the vaccines themselves were in limited supply, as both SII and Bharat Biotech were working on ramping up their production capacities.

India's digital divide came to the fore in these initial weeks.

Skilled individuals wrote applications and software robots to track available vaccination slots and block them quickly. The information was disseminated through mobile apps or social media and messaging platforms, like Telegram.[22]

For the first couple of months, there was a genuine concern that these technology aids working on top of CoWIN were leading to a skewed vaccine access. Those hoping to walk into the vaccination centres were unable to get any slots while those with access to technology could block slots as soon as they opened up for the coming days. This situation built up dissatisfaction and frustration in society, with a view being formed that technology was aiding a few while leaving a large chunk behind.[23]

The government had to act quickly on this feedback. In early May, about five weeks into the expanded vaccination drive that began on 1 April, the technology team behind CoWIN restricted the number of API calls that third-party applications could make to the CoWIN platform.[24] Technology innovation was not curtailed, but an attempt was made to prevent its misuse.

One major characteristic of any consumer-facing technology platform is that it becomes the zeitgeist of the underlying process it seeks to implement. CoWIN was no different in the evaluation it faced.

During the worst of the second wave of the pandemic in April and May 2021, vaccine enthusiasm also started to peak. When the virus started to devour thousands every day, there was a realization that vaccination was an important preventive tool. This led to a rush for vaccines at a time when the supply was gradually ramping up. In these months, the healthcare system itself was under tremendous strain, with understaffing and overburdened workers.

Even those individuals who were good with technology and could even use enabling tools, like Telegram bots, faced challenges in booking appointment slots for their vaccination. The blame for this rather complex situation fell on CoWIN.

A multivariate problem was oversimplified to a narrative that CoWIN does not work.

This narrative took even deeper roots when the central government decided to let states procure their own vaccines in April. However, coinciding with these couple of months, CoWIN became a deeper collateral casualty. The states also requested the central government to allow state-specific technology apps and not just rely on CoWIN. In a letter written to PM Modi, the Maharashtra CM Uddhav Thackeray requested that each state be allowed to develop its own app, and the data across states can be shared with the CoWIN platform.[25] The CM of Delhi, Arvind Kejriwal, made a similar request to then Health Minister Dr Harsh Vardhan.[26]

Several states, like Karnataka, Chhattisgarh and Punjab, started the process of developing their own apps.[27] One key perceived utility of state-specific apps was that each state could pick and choose what it considered 'priority groups'. They could decide the order in which potential beneficiaries would be vaccinated and this order could differ from the criteria that the central government had established for eligible groups.

India's Covid-19 response was constantly under the gaze of international media. The functioning of the CoWIN platform was no different. There were constant insinuations that the platform was a hindrance to the vaccination process. Throughout India's battle for getting over the travails of the pandemic, international media ensured that facts never came in the way of building an antagonistic narrative. The blame apportioned to CoWIN was no different.

One article claimed that Indians did not know how to use mobile apps and hence the pace of the vaccination was slow.[28] This allegation completely missed the fact that walk-in appointments were allowed from the very first day, where the user did not need to have technology proficiency to get vaccinated. Policy influencers from international not-for-profit sectors were liberally quoted to establish that the process had to be paper-based rather than digital. There was gratuitous advice about the need to remove phone number-linked tracking.

However, despite the internal and the external pressure to stop using CoWIN or at least limiting its use, the central government stood firm. It was evident that the platform was not to be crucified for the evolving nature of the vaccination ecosystem. In a supply-constrained environment, where vaccine manufacturing was still ramping up, hospitals had to balance between treating Covid-19 patients and vaccinating against the virus; healthcare professionals were working to the point of daily exhaustion and collapse, blaming the tracking and alleging that the monitoring technology was not ideal.

If states would have created their own apps, there could have been additional problems in terms of synchronizing data with CoWIN and potential problems of mutual recognition of state apps within the country itself. All CoWIN certificates had the same design, layout, information, etc. Hence, they were easier to verify through a single and simple application, even visually. If different states created their own systems, the certificates would have all looked different and would have contained different details.

However, with states unable to procure vaccines on their own—which was hardly surprising, as no company had extra stocks of vaccine—the debate over app proliferation also died down. Eventually, the push in the media against CoWIN, too, vanished. In hindsight, while health is a state subject, having a centralized tracking and monitoring platform like CoWIN worked best for the Indian vaccination programme.[29]

Data Beats Narratives

Sunlight is the best disinfectant. Data reverberates like the best thunderclaps.

While CoWIN was not competing for any commercial

recognition, a contrast with how the Big Tech platforms have grown is instructive. CoWIN effectively became the fastest tech platform globally to amass 200 million registrations in less than four months.[30] Typically, a globally successful Big Tech-led social media platform would take a year to hit 100 million users.

The CoWIN platform routinely handled more than a billion visits daily at the peak of the vaccination process.[31] The highest number of hits recorded in a day were 310 crore or 3.1 billion across all categories of users. The platform handled 1.37 crore or 13.7 million registrations within eight hours of the vaccination process opening for those in the age bracket of 18–44.

CoWIN gathered minimum data after mobile number registration. It collected data like name, age and gender. There were no breaches of security reported despite the scale at which it operated.

On 17 September 2021, on the PM's birthday, almost 2.5 crore or 25 million vaccine doses were administered in a single day. This number was more than the entire population of all but 54 countries in the world. Administering 25 million doses in 24 hours meant 3,000 doses per second. CoWIN platform quite gracefully handled this volume without any glitches. The platform scaled up beautifully, an apt symbol of true Indian resilience and the ability to adapt over time to meet tough challenges.

By the end of the year 2021, India administered 145 crore vaccine doses. Each of them was recorded on CoWIN. Each of them could be verified using CoWIN functionality for scanning Quick Response or QR codes on the certificates. Indian ingenuity worked, authoritatively so. The digital-first and mobile-first approach India adopted was handsomely vindicated.

Fantabulous Meets Surreal

The controversies around CoWIN moved from functional to rhetorical. One such controversy was about PM Modi's picture on the Indian vaccination certificates. There were numerous objections raised in the political and the opinion-making domain about how these pictures were not appropriate.

In May 2021, when the states had brief control over the vaccination process, Chhattisgarh and Jharkhand decided to remove[32] PM Modi's picture from the vaccine certificate. These states put the pictures of their respective CMs on the certificate. If the argument was not to have a picture on the vaccine certificate, replacing one picture with another would not really address the issue. Nonetheless, this measure occupied the narrative mindshare for a few weeks until the central government took over the vaccination process again in June.

Later in the year, Peter Myaliparambil, an RTI activist and one of the Kerala state coordinators of the National Campaign for the People's Right to Information, filed a public interest litigation (PIL) that the photograph of the PM on the vaccination certificate was an intrusion of his privacy.

This PIL came up for hearing in front of the single-judge bench of the Kerala high court of Justice P.V. Kunhikrishnan. He dismissed the plea as a frivolous petition and also added, 'I have a strong doubt that there is a political agenda also to the petitioner.'[33] He imposed a fine of ₹1 lakh on the petitioner for bringing up this frivolous petition and noted that it was the citizens' duty to respect the office of the PM of the country.[34]

Extending the Hand of Friendship

CoWIN was a winner and the platform ensured that India's vaccination process remained scientific, evidence-based and with real-time control. To showcase this achievement at a time when developed countries were struggling to run their paper-based processes, India organized a CoWIN Global Conclave. This conclave took place on 5 July 2021 and was attended by representatives of 142 countries. These included government officials as well as sector experts.

PM Modi inaugurated this virtual conference. It was yet another step to showcase Indian technological achievements to the world. He said, 'We have developed a robust, inclusive and scalable system that can prevent rent-seeking, black marketing and other malpractices.'[35]

Dr Harsh Vardhan, then health minister, remarked:

> Just recently in India, we marked the completion of six years of our Digital India initiative. A brainchild of our visionary Prime Minister Shri Narendra Modi Ji, various endeavors under the initiative have been helping us transform the lives of 1.37 billion plus Indians, drastically improving access to welfare schemes & services, plugging leakages and ensuring equitable access to growth & progress for one and all. Financial inclusion, furthering innovation & entrepreneurship, e-learning, health for all are just a few areas where giant strides have been made with the help of technology.
>
> In my humble opinion, CoWIN is the crown jewel of our Digital India initiative. This platform shall go down in history for facilitating inoculation of a large percentage of the world's population with ease, while simultaneously ensuring complete transparency. The accolades the platform has been winning globally and the interest expressed by so many partner nations in seeking our technology, expertise & know-how in this domain just reaffirms my belief.[36]

Following this conference, the Ministry of External Affairs offered the platform to any country that was in need of such a system as a global digital good. The CoWIN team of Ram Sewak Sharma created comprehensive documentation for the system, such that it could be used as an open source platform by any country in need.[37]

They Mocked, They Ignored, They Laughed, Then CoWIN

As the CoWIN platform stabilized, the criticism from the early months started turning into praise. The technological leverage that India deployed in negotiating mutual recognition of vaccine certificates with various countries also demonstrated how the platform had proven to be critical. With every single detail about the vaccine administered to every user captured on the certificate, there really was no way for other countries to question the veracity of Indian documentation. Even domestically, the ease of vaccination certificate access and the quick, app-based storage and download option converted the compulsive contrarians as well as professional pessimists into acknowledging the benefits of the technology-driven approach.

The United Nations Developed Programme paid a fitting tribute to the Indian vaccination programme and to CoWIN.

> To put it in perspective, India has administered more than 1.53 billion doses, more than the combined total achieved by the US, Brazil, Indonesia and Japan; only China has higher numbers (according to data available as of March 2022). The speed of administering those doses has been impressive – from 100 million to one billion from April to November 2021- an average of 3.75 million doses daily [...]
>
> One critical enabler of India's progress is a digital platform called CoWIN (Winning over Covid-19), developed by the government. It is a cloud-based system that facilitates registration, immunizations and appointments, and issues digital vaccine certificates.[38]

The power of CoWIN was demonstrated in a unique manner on 20 July 2022. The system had a record of all vaccinators who had contributed in the success of India's uphill vaccination battle.

Leveraging this structured information, PM Modi wrote a letter to every vaccinator registered on CoWIN, acknowledging their efforts when India hit the 2-billion (200-crore) mark of vaccinations administered.

His letter read:

> With your active participation, India has scripted history, yet again!
>
> Our journey of Covid vaccination started on 16th January 2021 and on 17th July 2022, we reached another significant milestone. It was a memorable day for the country as we completed administering 200 crore vaccine doses, an outstanding achievement in our fight against Covid-19.
>
> Saving lives in crucial, especially during a once-in-a-century global pandemic. Our vaccinators, healthcare workers, healthcare support staff and frontline workers have played a critical role in protecting Indians. This is a laudable example of dedication to duty and delivering when it is most necessary.
>
> From coldest mountains to the hottest deserts, from faraway villages to dense forests, the Covid-19 Vaccination Programme has left none behind and showed that New India excels in last mile delivery. The scale and speed that India imparted to the world's largest vaccination programme have been spectacular and this has happened due to the efforts of people like you.
>
> On this historic occasion, I applaud your contribution to India's COVID-19 Vaccination Programme and appreciate you for being at the forefront of such a crucial, life-saving mission.
>
> The achievement of 200 crore vaccine doses showcases the strength of the democratic, compassionate and service-oriented ethos of our Nation. The story of India's courage to deliver during a crisis will be cherished by generations to come.
>
> My best wishes to you and your family!
>
> Jai Hind![39]

Future Possibilities

CoWIN will evolve over time to adapt to other use cases too, wherever there is a large-scale mismatch between demand and supply. The government agencies involved in the design of the platform will work towards adapting it for helping out with blood and organ donations, and the operation of blood banks. This is an evolving area, and not just India but other countries may also benefit from India's innovation.[40]

India demonstrated that it was possible to assume technological leadership and create public health solutions, which stood apart not just in Indian history but also on the global stage.

In his tour to Silicon Valley in September 2015, PM Modi very passionately remarked, 'In this digital age, we have an opportunity to transform the lives of people in ways that were hard to imagine just a couple of decades ago. I see technology as a means to empower and as a tool that bridges the distance between hope and opportunity.'[41]

India realized this vision six years later, combating a crisis of a lifetime. The power of Digital India was proven when it was most required.

15

VASUDHAIVA KUTUMBAKAM

अयंनिजःपरोवेतिगणनालघुचेतसाम् ।
उदारचरितानांतुवसुधैवकुटुम्बकम् ।।

Ayam Nijah Paro Veti Ganana Laghucetasam
Udaracaritanam Tu Vasudhaiva Kutumbakam

Chapter 6 of the Maha Upanishad, one of the texts that deal with the philosophy and ontological knowledge of the Sanatana Dharma, carries this verse.[1]

It literally means: those with narrow minds think of people as relatives or strangers. One should be magnanimous in conduct, for the world is one family. This phrase is also inscribed in the Indian Parliament,[2] which can be seen as one proceeds from gate no. 1 to the central hall, reminding Indian lawmakers regularly of this ancient wisdom. As the pandemic paralysed country after country, it was clear that the world would have to face this challenge together. This was not just about providing moral support or strength to other nations. Real solutions were required, where those with the resources had to help those without access or sufficient resources to arrange for access.

India's embrace of *Vasudhaiva Kutumbakam* (the world is one family), in letter and spirit, became the defining motif of the country's international conduct. While India had been building a reputation as the 'pharmacy of the world', it had to stand true to that reputation when the tough test presented itself.

Through the course of the pandemic, it had become clear that it was far easier to practise multilateralism in the corridors of the UN than to adopt the comportment befitting the international postures countries presented. None of the multilateral bodies had come out as winners through their ingenuity and dynamism. The WHO, the nodal global agency to deal with the pandemic, was embattled through the course of the pandemic, despite late attempts at redeeming its role.

In this international scenario, individual countries had to take responsibility, not just for themselves but also for other countries in need. India showed that commitment and drive with great aplomb. In two ways, India's leadership at the global stage stood out through the crisis.

Vaccine Maitri: Vaccines for the World

India had committed very early on in the vaccine research and development cycle to making vaccines available to other countries. In his address to the seventy-fifth United Nations General Assembly session, PM Modi had remarked:

> Even during these very difficult times of a raging pandemic, the pharmaceutical industry of India has sent essential medicines to more than 150 countries. As the largest vaccine producing country of the world, I want to give one more assurance to the global community today, India's vaccine production and delivery capacity will be used to help all humanity in fighting this crisis. We are moving ahead with phase III clinical trials in India and in our neighbourhood. India will also help all the countries in enhancing their cold chain and storage capacities for the delivery of Vaccines.[3]

India was upfront about this commitment. It was a suo motu commitment made purely out of the conviction that the crisis needed collective resolve and cooperation.

The large global powers—the US, EU and UK—were looking to sign future contracts, similar to the financial market instruments. They would make advance payments to the main suppliers—Pfizer, Moderna and Janssen—for a committed capacity to be delivered later. Although this model did not work very smoothly for several buyers for a variety of reasons, this was the preferred way for the developed countries.

A feature in *The New York Times* referred to the behaviour of the developed countries as 'clearing the vaccine shelf'.[4]

They had all booked more doses than required to cover their entire population. In some cases like the US, the number of doses on which dibs was called exceeded the requirement for two doses for the entire population by an order of magnitude.

These powers had a similar model when it came to supporting vaccine access. The EU committed €300 million to the Gavi in June 2020.[5] Through that year, the financial commitments were indeed raised. This was, of course, significant and well-meaning support. But the main problem with this approach was that alliances, like Gavi and COVAX, became commercial buyers in a supply-constrained market.

When it came to competing commercially for vaccines for unknown future delivery dates, it was very difficult for global vaccine alliances and poorer countries to succeed against countries with big money. The cost of a single dose was the same, the value of every human life was the same, but those with deep pockets had effectively bought the first right to save who they wanted to using their purchasing power.

This situation would have put smaller countries and low- and middle-income countries in an awkward situation, where they would have had to struggle to get the necessary doses for their populations. In this context, India's position ameliorated the situation for a world that was stressed and stretched to its limits.

Dr Tedros Adhanom Ghebreyesus, director general of the WHO, praised India's commitment to the cause. In a telephonic conversation with PM Modi, he 'strongly appreciated Prime Minister Modi's unequivocal commitment to deploy India's capacities as a leading manufacturer of vaccines and pharmaceuticals for the benefit of humanity'.[6]

This inclusive approach was planned from the very outset. The thought process was very much in place even when it was not clear how many doses India would require. This thinking evolved in the early part of 2021. With the onset of the Delta wave in April, complete adult coverage became the accepted view and prescription. But the resolve to help those in need, starting with India's neighbourhood, was baked into the policy response as a first principle.

In October 2020, when the PM chaired one of the key meetings for reviewing the situation, he explicitly instructed officials to work on this aspect of engaging friendly countries on the topic of vaccine availability. He directed that India's efforts should not stay limited to the immediate neighbourhood but reach out to the entire world in providing vaccines, medicines and IT platforms for vaccine delivery systems.[7]

PM Modi also took this proposition directly to his counterparts and did not communicate only via envoys.

India and Bangladesh jointly commemorate Vijay Divas on 16 December to mark Bangladesh's freedom of 1971 from Pakistani occupation. In a summit meeting on 17 December with Sheikh Hasina, PM of Bangladesh, PM Modi assured her that vaccines would be made available to Bangladesh as and when produced in India.[8] The two leaders also acknowledged the research work being done by the scientists of both the countries. Indian scientists had been collaborating with their counterparts in other countries, including Afghanistan, Bangladesh, Bhutan, Maldives, Mauritius, Nepal and Sri Lanka, to strengthen their research capacities.[9]

Queries had started pouring in. Nepal requested Indian support in procuring 20 per cent of the total vaccine requirements.[10]

Bhutan and Qatar also showed interest in buying vaccines from India.[11]

India undertook extensive vaccine diplomacy and actively encouraged other countries to look at Indian vaccines as an option. The Ministry of External Affairs arranged for 64 foreign envoys to visit the facilities of Bharat Biotech and Biological E in December 2020.[12] The intent of this visit was to make the envoys aware of India's vaccine manufacturing capability and the ongoing research. The tour was organized jointly with the DBT and the BIRAC. The ambassadors and high commissioners of Australia, Denmark, Croatia, Sri Lanka, Bhutan and South Korea joined the visit.

Keeping the promise of treating the world as our own family, the deliveries of vaccines to other countries started on 21 January, five days after the vaccination programme began in India.[13]

India called its global outreach 'Vaccine Maitri'—literally meaning 'Vaccine Friendship'. Every package shipped was inscribed with the Tricolour and a Sanskrit saying: '*Sarve Santu Niramaya* (may no one suffer from illness).' This truly captured the spirit of the Indian intent and effort.

Bhutan became the first recipient of the Indian vaccines. On 20 January 2021, India sent 1.5 lakh vaccine doses to Bhutan,[14] which was also the first country that PM Modi had visited after taking the oath of office in 2014. This grant was supplemented in March with another 4 lakh vaccine doses.[15] A significant part of Bhutan's total population of 8 lakh could be covered with Indian grants.

Maldives was another country that received a vaccine grant on the same day. Maldives' President Ibrahim Mohamed Solih had been a longstanding friend of India and the two countries have enjoyed strong old ties. A grant of 1 lakh doses was sent on 20 January to Maldives, with a follow-up grant of another 1 lakh doses in February. Maldives also purchased Indian vaccines commercially, apart from receiving a COVAX allocation. About a quarter of Maldives' population was protected by Indian vaccines.[16]

On 21 January, India shipped 10 lakh vaccine doses to Nepal as the first grant. Through the year, Nepal also continued to buy vaccines commercially. Nepal became a big recipient of Indian vaccines from the COVAX facility. In total, Nepal received almost 95 lakh doses of Covishield.[17] Of these, 11 lakh doses were granted by India and the rest came via market mechanisms. The 95 lakh doses were sufficient to cover about one-sixth of Nepal's population of about 3 crore.

Bangladesh, the country with which there had been most extensive discussions on making Indian vaccines available, also received the first shipment for 20 lakh doses on 21 January. In total, Bangladesh received 33 lakh doses in grants over the year, 97.8 lakh doses from COVAX and directly purchased 1.5 crore doses from India. These 2.8 crore doses were sufficient to cover 8.4 per cent of Bangladesh's population of 16.6 crore.[18]

Myanmar, another important neighbour, was specifically promised vaccine access. The Indian Chief of Army Staff, General M.M. Naravane, and Foreign Secretary, Harsh Vardhan Shringla, in October 2020, discussed vaccine access in a diplomatic meet. The Foreign Secretary had indicated to the Myanmar government that India may consider prioritizing vaccines for the country.[19]

On 22 January, India complied. As many as 15 lakh Covishield doses were granted to Myanmar, followed by another 2 lakh Covaxin doses on 11 February. Over the year, India made a total grant of 37 lakh doses to the southeastern neighbour. Myanmar also bought 1.75 crore doses. The Made in India vaccines were enough to cover a quarter of Myanmar's population of 5.48 crore.[20]

On the same day, vaccines were sent to Mauritius and Seychelles. The former got a grant of 1 lakh vaccines and the latter, 50,000. Mauritius later also bought another 3 lakh doses, in total creating the ability to vaccinate one-sixth of its population with Made in India vaccines. Likewise, Seychelles, a small country with just about 1 lakh inhabitants, could cover almost a quarter of their population, administering Made in India vaccines.[21]

Sri Lanka, Bahrain and Oman were the other Asian countries where Made in India vaccines landed in the month of January.[22] But it wasn't just the Asian friends that India was engaging with.

On the evening of 22 January, Indian social media was taken by storm. The Brazilian President Jair Bolsonaro tweeted a thank you note to India and PM Modi for allowing exports of vaccines. Brazil bought 40 lakh doses from India. That this was an important gesture by a friendly country was visible in the image President Bolsonaro used in his post. He tweeted[23] an image of Lord Hanuman carrying vaccines from India to Brazil, recalling the event from the Ramayana, where Lord Hanuman fetched *sanjeevani booti* to save the life of Lakshmana, Lord Rama's younger brother. The tweet read:

> *Namaskar, Primeiro Ministro*
>
> *@narendramodi*
>
> *– O Brasil sente-se honrado em ter um grande parceiro para superar um obstáculo global. Obrigado por nos auxiliar com as exportações de vacinas da Índia para o Brasil.*
>
> *– Dhanyavaad!* धन्यवाद
>
> (Namaskar, Prime Minister
>
> @narendramodi
>
> Brazil feels honoured to have a great partner to overcome a global obstacle by joining efforts. Thank you for assisting us with the vaccines exports from India to Brazil.
>
> Thank you!)

Although 40 lakh doses were not big relative to Brazil's population, the presidential intervention demonstrated the goodwill India had generated by placing human lives on equal footing around the world. India also had a huge vaccine requirement, but it continued to engage with the rest of the world in the best possible manner under the circumstances. This sense of purpose, purity and sincerity of intent won India tremendous goodwill through the first quarter of 2021.

This expression of profound gratitude was further visible in February when India sent grants of Covishield to Barbados, Dominica and Dominican Republic.

The island nations in the Caribbean, part of the larger West Indies, have been best connected with India through their collective nomenclature. When Christopher Columbus landed on the island of Hispaniola—home to the Dominican Republic—he wrongly assumed he was in India. The name 'West Indies' thus created a permanent shared history with India.

On 9 February, when a plane landed carrying 1 lakh vaccines in Bridgetown, the Indian officials were welcomed by none other than Barbadian PM Mia Mottley, Foreign Minister Jerome Xavier Walcott and Health Minister Jeffrey Bostic.[24] The vaccines were given celebrity treatment—after all, in February 2021, the virus was still wreaking global havoc, and a small country, like Barbados, with a population of less than 3 lakh would have otherwise had to fight tooth and nail to get vaccines.

Barbados was faced with a large-scale outbreak[25] of Covid-19 around this time, which impacted their police forces and prison setup in a big way. This became a big political and national security issue in the country. In the face of this security situation, PM Mottley had reached out to various big countries for help.

PM Mottley wrote a letter to PM Modi just before Republic Day, seeking 2 lakh vaccines.[26] While the Indian government was still considering this request, an unseemly controversy broke out with respect to Barbados. The singer Rihanna—one of the best-known Barbadians globally—tweeted in support of farmers who had been protesting in New Delhi for many weeks after the government had enacted three agriculture farm laws. These protesters attacked Red Fort, a key national monument, on the Republic Day. While there was a great deal of anger within the country about this incident, an orchestrated international campaign was unleashed to put pressure on India, painting the aggressors as heroes and the government as villain. Rihanna's tweet[27] in this context generated a lot of anger within India.

Yet, such political considerations were not accounted for when the Indian government decided to respond to PM Mottley's request. Despite a discordant situation in the country, India stuck to the task of helping as many countries as possible.

PM Mottley tweeted soon after: 'India's gift of 100,000 COVID-19 vaccines arrived Barbados earlier today. This was a very special moment for all Barbadians and I want to thank Prime Minister Modi for his quick, decisive, and magnanimous action in allowing us to be the beneficiary of these vaccines.'[28]

Her admiration for the Indian effort did not stop here. In an additional gesture of gratitude, PM Mottley acknowledged India's helping hand in a supremely gracious and thoughtful manner. On 1 March, the day PM Modi took his vaccine and tweeted about it, she quoted on top of his tweet: 'PM Modi @narendramodi made it possible for more than 40K persons in Barbados and tens of thousands elsewhere, to receive their 1st dose of COVISHIELD via #VaccineMaitri before receiving his. A genuine demonstration of generosity. Thank you and we wish you continued good health.'[29]

This same warmth and bonding was visible in Dominica as well. The PM of Dominica, Roosevelt Skerrit, personally received the 70,000 vaccine doses that India had shipped. For a country of just 72,000 people, this was a big boost—half of the country could get fully vaccinated with the help of the doses supplied by India.

Early morning, PM Skerrit announced his country's vaccination drive with a solicitous acknowledgement:

'Good Morning to all Citizens and Residents,

'Our nation is ready to launch the largest vaccination campaign in modern history as we have received 70,000 doses of the COVID-19 vaccine from India.'[30]

Later the same evening, he put out a commemorative video on his Twitter feed with the caption: 'Even though I trust every word of the bible, I must confess that I did not imagine that the prayers of my country would have been answered so swiftly. Thank You India. @narendramodi.'[31]

He then made a televised statement to his country, yet again profusely praising the Indian gesture. PM Skerrit said:

> I must confess that I did not imagine that the prayers of my country would have been answered so swiftly. Being the leader of a small Caribbean island of a population of 72,000 people, I did not fancy my chances of getting such a swift positive response to my request of India's Prime Minister Narendra Modi. One would have thought and understood that in a global pandemic such as this, a nation's size and might would have been the primary considerations. But it is to the credit of Prime Minister Modi that our request was considered on merit and the equality of our people was recognized. I would like to take this opportunity once again to express my heartfelt thanks and appreciation to Prime Minister Modi, his government and the citizens of India.[32]

These expressions from the leaders of Barbados and the Commonwealth of Dominica really captured the essence of Vaccine Maitri. India stood up for friends around the world, in many cases making sure that a sizable portion of those countries' population got covered by two doses of vaccine. Vaccinating several other countries in parallel to one's own citizens was a selfless gesture, which no other country in the world could lay an easy claim to.

Several other Caribbean countries were soon covered. On 27 February, Saint Lucia (with population of 1.9 lakh) received 25,000 doses of Covishield vaccine, Saint Kitts and Nevis (with population of 53,000), 20,000 doses, Saint Vincent and the Grenadines (with population of 1.2 lakh), 40,000 doses, Antigua and Barbuda (with population of 1 lakh), 40,000 doses, and the

Republic of Suriname (with population of 6 lakh) received 50,000 doses. All of these were supplied as grants.[33]

In the General Council meeting held in early March at the World Trade Organization (WTO), the representative of Saint Lucia took the floor to acknowledge India's stupendous role. The statement made on behalf of the Caribbean Community or CARICOM, an intergovernmental organization with a membership of 15 countries, said:

> All CARICOM countries had signed on to the highly valued and much appreciated COVAX Facility which would provide up to 20% of Members' needs. That limited supply however would not allow them to attain regional herd immunity that was necessary to kickstart the durable recovery. CARICOM thanked the Governments of India and South Africa and the African Union for their generosity and solidarity during that time. The Government of India, through the generosity of Prime Minister Narendra Modi had donated an initial installment of 170,000 vaccines to Barbados and Dominica through bilateral arrangement. CARICOM thanked its Member States Barbados and Dominica for having shared the initial supplies from India with the rest of the Caribbean Community.
>
> CARICOM reported that the Indian Government had dispatched an additional 175,000 vaccines to five CARICOM Member States. That act of selflessness was testament to the stalwart solidarity of the Government and People of India with CARICOM. The Republic of South Africa and the African Union had also carved out an allocation of vaccines for CARICOM countries through the African Union's African Medical Supplies Platform. CARICOM urged vaccine producing countries to exercise due restraint in imposing export restrictions on COVID-19 vaccines. No country was truly protected unless all countries were equally

> protected. CARICOM also implored all countries to work on improving trade logistics to enhance the timely delivery of and access to vaccines.[34]

In the month of March, the focus shifted to the African nations. About 40 African countries received the Made in India vaccines by April. India also prioritized the need for UN peacekeeping and UN healthcare workers in the first few months of 2021.

By the time the deadly Delta wave hit India in April 2021, the Made in India vaccines had reached almost 95 different countries and entities, including UN bodies. India had made sure that low- and middle-income countries, which would otherwise not have had any chance to procure any vaccine at all, were prioritized at the same level as Indians themselves.

Vaccine exports resumed after India's own vaccination drive had been successfully completed. In 2022, the Novavax vaccine also started being shipped under various brand names. The Quad initiative for providing vaccines to the countries in the Indo-Pacific region also scaled up with the initial consignments of vaccines going to Thailand and Cambodia.

Another feather in the cap of India's manufacturing came in July 2022. The SII got the US FDA nod to export Novavax's vaccines to the US.[35] This was the fourth vaccine approved for Covid-19 in the US and it would be labelled as Made in India under the partnership arrangement of the two companies.

On 3 July, India exported 32.43 lakh or 3.243 million doses of the Novavax vaccine to the US.[36] Novavax supplies added countries like Australia, the Netherlands, New Zealand and the US from the developed world as the export destinations for Made in India vaccines.

By the end of October 2022, India had exported close to 27 crore or 270 million vaccine doses to 100 countries.[37] It was not just the numbers. Three things stood out from the Vaccine Maitri programme.

First, the way India embraced the world demonstrated that the country held the lives of its neighbouring nations as well as many friendly countries at par with human lives in India. Actions are the real testament to one's character. The Indian focus was to act, not just make empty promises.

Second, the help extended by India covered a reasonable proportion of the population in many countries. The quantities supplied to several countries were enough to cover vulnerable sections in their territory. This helped stabilize the spread of the pandemic in these countries.

Third, India neither hoarded vaccines nor acted unreasonably in sharing what it had. Indian grants and sales had no strings attached when it came to the transfer of vaccines. To deal with the large western pharmaceutical firms, small countries would have had to provide sovereign guarantees. To a practical extent, the Indian position ameliorated this situation for those who we call our friends.

Vaccine Trilemma: An Intellectual Property Battle

Intellectual property rights (IPR) form a key aspect of global trade and business architecture. Intellectual property rights have fuelled innovation and ensured that capital gets deployed in commercializing these innovations. The global commercial protection available to inventors, designers, artists and practically anyone with a creative streak has been an underwriting mechanism for the investment of time, effort, mental faculties and money in pursuit of excellence.

The history of intellectual property goes back several centuries. In 1421, architect and engineer, Filippo Brunelleschi, received the first-ever industrial patent in Florence, Italy, which enabled him to manufacture special barges to transport marble.[38] This patent allowed him three-year exclusivity on this product.

IPR—encompassing patents, trademarks and copyright—

evolved differently in different countries since. While their importance was well understood, there were no international standards for a long time. Every country had a different approach, and cross-border intellectual property protection was difficult, if not outright impossible. This situation was not a big impediment in a world that was globalized only through colonization and not through shared interests and values.

However, as national borders began to be drawn, redrawn, crossed and traversed, the recognition that such IPR were important in a global context became stronger. In 1883, the Paris Convention, for the first time, ensured that there was some degree of international homogenization of the ideas that formed the basis of these rights.[39] Paris was followed by Berne and Madrid Conventions and by the turn of the twentieth century, the world of business had a reasonably common understanding of this subject.

In fact, the international collaboration in the area of IPR predates even the League of Nations. One of the first of its kind, the United International Bureaux for the Protection of Intellectual Property (BIRPI) was an international organization that was set up in 1893. It administered the Berne Convention for the Protection of Literary and Artistic Works and the Paris Convention for the Protection of Industrial Property. This organization was originally set up in Berne but moved to Geneva, the global hub of multilateralism, in 1960.

In 1967, the World Intellectual Property Organization Convention established the World Intellectual Property Organization (WIPO) in Geneva, which became the successor to the BIRPI. Today, the WIPO is the global forum for intellectual property services, policy, information and cooperation.[40]

While the WIPO worked on framework and policies, there had to be a mechanism to make IPR available in a world where complexity and interconnectivity were increasing exponentially with every passing decade. That role was fulfilled by the WTO, the successor to the General Agreement on Tariff and Trade, established on 1 January 1995.

In the extensive discussions covering all aspects of global trade preceding the formation of the WTO, intellectual property was also a key element. These discussions, known as the Uruguay Round, went on for nine years starting in 1986. The Agreement on Trade-Related Aspects of Intellectual Property Rights (TRIPS) became the most comprehensive international agreement ever signed to enforce the concept of IPR since the concept came into the picture in 1421. The WTO and the WIPO have worked closely since then.

The TRIPS Agreement covers five broad areas:

- How general provisions and basic principles of the multilateral trading system apply to international intellectual property
- What the minimum standards of protection are for intellectual property rights that members should provide
- Which procedures members should provide for the enforcement of those rights in their own territories
- How to settle disputes on intellectual property between members of the WTO
- Special transitional arrangements for the implementation of TRIPS provisions.[41]

The agreement on the TRIPS was seen as crucial in protecting new capital investments towards research and development. This is because the agreement has served two purposes. First, the agreement defines minimum substantive standards of protection available to the rights holders of various types of intellectual property. Second, the agreement also establishes the procedures through which the rights holders can enforce their rights in a meaningful manner. This dual characteristic has made this agreement a cornerstone of modern-day business innovation.

But should there be any limitations on IPR? What happens when the world is in the throes of an unprecedented pandemic?

Can there be any exceptions and if yes, when should they be made?

The agreement tries to answer these questions. Part II—Standards Concerning the Availability, Scope and Use of Intellectual Property Rights of the agreement defines both the protection available as well as exceptions for various types of IPR. Under Section 5, which addresses patent as a type of IPR, Article 31 of the agreement titled 'Other Use without Authorization of the Right Holder' addresses exceptional circumstances.

Article 31 allows use of IPR without the express authorization of rights holders but is subject to a fairly stringent set of conditionalities that need to be met. In fact, the article lists 12 conditions to be met, with the twelfth condition leading to three additional enforcement requirements.[42] In general, these conditions have been tough to meet, especially in the case of pharmaceuticals, which is a very complex process-manufacturing industry.

Clause (f) of the Article 31 states that 'any such use shall be authorized predominantly for the supply of the domestic market of the Member authorizing such use'. This causes an additional problem in the case of pharmaceuticals. The countries most impacted by a devastating disease may not be the ones best equipped to exceptionally authorize the use of the flexibilities of Article 31 to remedy the situation. And the country using these flexibilities is expected to substantially use the provision for the domestic market, not for exports.

This logistical issue first faced the world at the turn of the century. Much before the Covid-19 pandemic, the world faced the scourge of acquired immunodeficiency syndrome or AIDS caused by the human immunodeficiency virus or HIV. As AIDS ravaged several parts of the world in the decade of the '90s in the last century, there were concerns that there would be no pharmaceutical interventions available to fight or at least reduce the impact of the killer disease.

This is when the WTO members from Africa proposed that the TRIPS Agreement should be amended. The Ministerial

Declaration of the Doha Conference of the WTO, held in November 2001, made for momentous reading:

> We agree that the TRIPS Agreement does not and should not prevent Members from taking measures to protect public health. Accordingly, while reiterating our commitment to the TRIPS Agreement, we affirm that the Agreement can and should be interpreted and implemented in a manner supportive of WTO Members' right to protect public health and, in particular, to promote access to medicines for all.[43]

A process was set in motion to realize this Doha Declaration on the TRIPS Agreement and Public Health. Any WTO agreement can only be amended with the concurrence of two-thirds of the membership as stipulated in Paragraph 3 of the Article X of the Marrakesh Agreement establishing the WTO.[44] This long process to bring in more flexibility in the use of the TRIPS Agreement came to a conclusion in 2017.

In the Council for Trade-Related Aspects of Intellectual Property Rights meeting held on 30 January 2017 in Geneva, the chairperson noted that as of 23 January, the necessary number of instruments accepting the protocol modifying the TRIPS Agreement had been received.[45] Thus, the agreement was modified. This resulted in the introduction of Article 31bis in the agreement, which among other provisions, also made it possible for countries exercising flexibility in using IPR to export goods thus produced to other countries.

This 'African Amendment' was perhaps the best example of a pro-development agenda prevailing in the WTO, otherwise perceived as dominated by the rich, developed world.

In 2020, a natural question that arose was, can the provisions of 'compulsory licensing' that were now possible within the TRIPS Agreement be used for Covid-19 vaccines? The question became increasingly critical as the vaccine trilemma unravelled.

Access, equity and affordability were the three key dimensions of vaccine administration for any country. It was clear that until all three dimensions were optimized, no country would be able to cover a significant part of its population—a prerequisite to controlling the pandemic. The news of vaccine trials, successes and disappointments were keenly followed around the world. Then reality sunk in—it was increasingly clear that while the vaccine excitement may be global, the vaccine trilemma was local. It was left to individual countries to fend for themselves and try and tick as many boxes as possible. More and more countries realized that they were not able to address one, two or all three of these dimensions. Some countries had no way to access vaccines at all. Others were mired in moral conflicts on how to distribute limited supplies of vaccines in the best possible way in the light of eager and willing consumption demand. Others were made to sign usurious contracts, staking their sovereignty to private pharmaceutical firms to get vaccines.[46]

Article 31bis was also deemed insufficient due to the specificity of the process of implementation. The article may work for compulsory licensing of a small, localized emergency situation. But it would have been very difficult to implement it in the way Covid-19 merited a response.

A South Centre—an organization based in Geneva, which promotes global south cooperation—research paper brought out these frailties:

> Empirical evidence demonstrates that the system is so cumbersome that the generic pharmaceutical industry has considered that the system is unworkable. Indeed, to use the system, potential generic or biosimilar manufacturers would have to make considerable investment of resources and time to develop a limited quantity of products [...] The products developed by them under the system cannot be redirected to supplying any other market should such an event occur.[47]

This is where India and South Africa took the lead to catalyse a global discussion on the severity of the pandemic and the need to think and implement radical, not just incremental solutions. The two countries got together in mid-2020, anticipating the vaccine trilemma much in advance, to work towards a TRIPS waiver for Covid-19-related goods.

The TRIPS Waiver

The key idea was that the provisions of the agreement itself should be suspended in entirety to promote the manufacturing of Covid-related goods, such as diagnostics, therapeutics and vaccines in multiple locations around the world. This was an unconventional idea from the standpoint of the WTO, known generally for defiant stodginess. It was also sure to tick off the developed countries as well as the supremely strong global pharmaceutical lobbies.

Even before the proposal could go to the WTO, an extensive internal consultation by the government was undertaken. Brajendra Navnit, an IAS officer of the Tamil Nadu cadre from 1999, had just taken over in Geneva as India's ambassador and permanent representative to the WTO in June 2020.[48] A young and dedicated officer with a proven track record, including that of working in the PMO for over five years, Navnit helmed the process of creating internal support for this proposal.

Long discussions ensued between Geneva and New Delhi. Thorough analysis was conducted on the merits of the proposal. Various possibilities were thrashed out in these discussions, including planning for potential reactions of the developed countries. One strand of thought was that this proposal may lead to adverse events in other ongoing WTO negotiations. These possibilities were discussed in minutiae, with the Minister of Commerce and Industry Piyush Goyal leading the analysis and the plan to gather support for such a proposal.[49]

On their part, South Africa also undertook a similar exercise. Eventually both the countries agreed that the grave pandemic situation demanded such a step.

Indian officials in Geneva also undertook extensive consultations there to apprise other members of such a proposal. Socialization of the proposal in Geneva was critical. The WTO worked on consensus, and the Geneva-based officials of various countries would be able to take the message back to their respective capitals. The WHO is also located in Geneva, home to several UN bodies. It was the natural base for canvassing support from civil society and organizations working on global health issues. The Indian officials conducted more than 100 meetings in Geneva before and after the introduction of the waiver proposal to build support.[50]

On 2 October 2020, on the occasion of Gandhi Jayanti, India and South Africa jointly communicated their proposal to the Council for Trade-Related Aspects of Intellectual Property Rights. The four-page document titled 'Waiver from Certain Provisions of the TRIPS Agreement for the Prevention, Containment and Treatment of Covid-19—Communication from India and South Africa' stated:

> In these exceptional circumstances, we request that the Council for TRIPS recommends, as early as possible, to the General Council a waiver from the implementation, application and enforcement of Sections 1, 4, 5, and 7 of Part II of the TRIPS Agreement in relation to prevention, containment or treatment of COVID-19.
>
> The waiver should continue until widespread vaccination is in place globally, and the majority of the world's population has developed immunity hence we propose an initial duration of [x] years from the date of the adoption of the waiver.
>
> We request that the Council for TRIPS urgently recommends to the General Council adoption of the annexed decision text.[51]

The proposal was very clear. The world needed to take note of the gravity of the situation. The limitations of the TRIPS Agreement had to be sidestepped to ensure that the world could hope to defeat Covid-19.

The proposal came up for the first discussion on 15 October at the scheduled meeting of the Council for Trade-Related Aspects of Intellectual Property Rights. By this time, Kenya and Eswatini had already agreed to co-sponsor the proposal, which was introduced by South Africa on the floor of the WTO.

It was a very powerful intervention that opened with a clear recognition of the problem and the need to relook at the applicability of the IPR in the circumstances. South Africa opened the statement with:

> I have the honour to introduce this proposal on behalf of the delegations of Eswatini, India, Kenya and South Africa.
>
> The COVID-19 pandemic is a clarion call for us to answer to the better angels of our nature. High-minded language on solidarity and global public goods, however, has not been matched by tangible steps to share know-how and intellectual property rights to facilitate deep technology transfer in the COVID-19 response. Business as usual approaches will not bring back the countless lives that were lost, neither will it ensure that IP barriers to the prevention, containment and treatment of COVID-19 will be addressed effectively.[52]

The Indian statement was delivered by Gurleen Kaur, the youngest member of the Indian contingent in Geneva. An officer of the Indian Foreign Service, Kaur made an impassioned plea to the trade mandarins of the world:

> We thank South Africa for its detailed and comprehensive statement. We also thank UNAIDS, UNITAID, MSF, other academics, researchers as well as numerous civil society

organizations who have expressed widespread support for our proposal.

Let me also take this opportunity to thank the Secretariat for its report on the TRIPS Agreement and COVID-19. We believe that it is not merely coincidental that this report came out the day before, more than six months into the COVID-19 pandemic. At least our proposal could generate enough interest for action now. However, in our view, the measures listed in the report are not sufficient for an effective COVID-19 response, which necessitates the need for our waiver proposal.

At the outset we would like to emphasize that this proposal is particularly important to cater for those who have insufficient or no manufacturing capacities in the health products required to combat the COVID crisis. In the past few months, India has supplied medical products and equipment needed in fighting the pandemic to more than 150 countries and resisted the attempts to corner the supplies by a few countries. We would like to remind the Members that in a global pandemic where every country is affected, we need a global solution. And our waiver proposal represents an open and expedited global solution to allow uninterrupted collaboration in development, production and supply of health products and technologies required for an effective COVID-19 response.

South Africa has very clearly explained the purpose and objective of our proposal. In this regard, we want to highlight following points:

First, there can be no denying the fact that the development of and equitable access to the tools—such as diagnostics, therapeutics, treatments, vaccines etc.—required to fight the COVID-19 pandemic are limited by IP barriers. It is quite evident from an array of lawsuits filed by private companies in different parts of the world for IP infringement on COVID-19 products. In the past few months, we have also seen that IPRs do come in the way of scaling up production of test kit reagents, ventilator valves, N95 respirators, therapeutics, fluorescent proteins and other technologies used in development of vaccines etc.

Second, governments across the globe are supporting development of new health technologies, in particular vaccines by pouring billions of USD of public funds into research and development. The EU tracker of pledged resources for access to tests, treatments and vaccines stands at EUR 16 billion. Therefore, the often-repeated argument that monopoly rights are needed to allow the inventors to recoup their investment does not seem to apply in case of development of health products and technologies required for handling the ongoing COVID-19 crisis.

Third, we have heard from some Members in the previous meetings that voluntary licenses are the most appropriate solution to scale up manufacturing in response to COVID-19. However, the fact remains that not a single IP holder has shown willingness to commit to the COVID-19 Technology Access Pool (C-TAP) and the ACT-Accelerator voluntary initiatives launched under the aegis of WHO. In fact, the representative from WHO in the Council admitted in response to a question that no pharmaceutical company has committed to sharing its IP and technologies in the C-TAP pool since its launch more than five months ago. Given the refusal by the pharmaceutical industry to routinely offer nonexclusive licenses with worldwide coverage to facilitate global access, clearly the solution to ending the pandemic does not lie in voluntary licenses.

Fourth, with regard to existing flexibilities under the TRIPS Agreement, the same are not adequate to address the fast-changing landscape of COVID-19. Of particular concern for countries with insufficient or no manufacturing capacity is Article 31bis, which is limited to pharmaceutical products, and was not designed to address challenges arising from pandemics of this scale and magnitude. Medical devices like ventilators, dialysis machines etc. that are crucial for combating the ongoing pandemic, may not be covered under the scope of Article 31bis. There is a reason why the Special Compulsory Licensing system has been used only once. Requirements under this System that exporters and importers have to comply with, are extremely onerous and time-consuming, thereby rendering it of no practical utility towards handling the ongoing pandemic.

Fifth, we have included four sections of the TRIPS Agreement, namely patents, copyrights, industrial designs and undisclosed information or trade secrets, in our proposal. This is because the health products and technologies like test kits, masks, medicines, vaccines, components of ventilators like valves, control mechanisms and the algorithms and CAD files used in their manufacturing are protected by these four types of IPRs. This ensures that our waiver proposal does not suggest a waiver from all TRIPS obligations, but only from these specific sections and that too only to the extent the same are essential for effective handling of the COVID-19 crisis.

Sixth, it may be noted that the waivers granted to LDC Members with respect to obligations in Article 70.8 and 70.9 and their rights under Article 66.1 of the TRIPS Agreement are in no way impacted by this proposal.

Lastly, we want to clarify that the time period of 'X' years does not signify that we are seeking a waiver for an indefinite duration. The actual waiver duration will be negotiated and be limited to a period that this Council finds necessary to effectively handle the COVID crisis. Furthermore, the waiver will be reviewed annually by the General Council in accordance with the provisions of Article IX (4) of the WTO

> Agreement. We are flexible with regard to the scope and duration of the waiver. We look forward to constructively engaging with Members having any questions or concerns regarding our proposal.
>
> We believe that now is the time for WTO as an organization to rise up to the collective call for defeating the pandemic. It will not succeed in its efforts in rebuilding the COVID affected economies unless it acts now to first save those lives that are going to build these economies. It's time for Members to take collective responsibility and put people's lives before anything else. History will not judge us kindly if we do not act immediately to save large scale loss of human life and health and allow global dysfunction to prevail over global cooperation. We hope that Members will support our proposal that will ensure that vaccines and treatments become truly global public goods.[53]

India had taken the lead on the global stage to combat a common global threat. It demonstrated the foresight in explaining that the market mechanisms by themselves were not going to be sufficient to deliver the vaccine trilemma of access, equity and affordability. It would require express intergovernmental cooperation and intervention.

India's concerns and the foresight were to be proven right over time. The American pharmaceutical giant Pfizer made nearly $37 billion in sales in 2021 from its blockbuster Covid-19 vaccine.[54] Moderna, the maker of the other successful mRNA vaccine, clocked $18.5 billion in revenue in 2021, most of which came from the vaccine.[55] The company had made $803 million in revenue in the previous year, marking a nearly 23-times jump year-on-year.

In March 2021, the Norwegian ambassador to the WTO, Dagfinn Sørli, took over the chairmanship of the Council for Trade-Related Aspects of Intellectual Property Rights. He proposed a text-based negotiation process on the proposal put forward by India and South Africa. The WTO members would make written submissions and the council would hope to arrive at a common consensus.

The negotiations in the council carried on through the year in the run up to the flagship event of the WTO in November 2021, dubbed the Ministerial Conference. The twelfth edition of the Ministerial Conference was expected to take a decision on the TRIPS waiver in Geneva. With persistent efforts of the delegations of India and South Africa, the waiver proposal continued to gain support widely. Eventually, over 2021, more than 60 members came together to support the proposal. This included a long list of countries willing to put their name against a precedent-creating step on management of global intellectual property.

Meanwhile, the US saw a change in the government after the election held in November 2020. As the new president took over in January 2021, one of the key decisions taken by the regime in the first few months was to back the proposed TRIPS waiver. The language was cautious, stating[56] that the US was willing to participate in the text-based negotiation process at the WTO to arrive at a conclusion of the waiver discussions. The WTO makes decisions by consensus. To arrive at a multilateral consensus, it is important that the key trade actors back a proposal. The US lending its support, however cautious, was an important sign for the other members.

However, right from the outset, three key members of the WTO—the EU, the UK and Switzerland—continued to oppose the TRIPS waiver. Their key contention was that the waiver was not really required to expand the production of Covid-19 goods around the world. There were other equivalent methods, including increased use of trade as a lever.

While the proposal made by India and South Africa covered all Covid-19 goods, the spotlight got fixed largely on the vaccines over the year 2021. With most countries having experienced a minimum of two waves of the pandemic, the need for vaccines was clear and uncontested.

When the proponents of the waiver pointed out that trade as a lever for vaccines would not solve the problem of affordability, the opponents of the waiver did not quite address the challenge directly. They continued to repeat the same arguments in the Council for Trade-Related Aspects of Intellectual Property Rights that waiver was a subpar instrument. They characterized the waiver as a sledgehammer technique to solve what, in their opinion, was a relatively manageable problem. The developing world and the Global South continued to contest this view with alacrity and growing frustration throughout 2021.

Some of the opponents of the waiver also continued to push for compulsory licensing using the flexibility imparted by the Article 31bis. Unfortunately, these opponents failed to appreciate—or chose not to appreciate under the influence of their domestic pharmaceutical lobbies—that the Article 31bis was a targeted solution. It would work between specific pairs of members for specific drugs in a defined timeframe. The problem posed by the Covid-19 pandemic was significantly wider and deeper than the typical scenarios envisaged to be solved by the design of Article 31bis.

India continued to stress in the negotiations that as far as vaccines were concerned, it was the net giver of intellectual property. India had Covaxin and the DNA-based vaccine of Zydus Cadila, which had been approved by the Indian regulators in August 2021. As far as diagnostics and therapeutics were concerned, India again had domestic production of many items, which would fall under the ambit of the proposed waiver.

A big blow was dealt to the negotiation process when the WTO had to postpone the Ministerial Conference in Geneva in November 2021. With the global outbreak of the Omicron variant-led wave of Covid-19, the organization had to take a tough call, based on the guidance of the Swiss authorities. This postponement of the Ministerial Conference sucked the wind out of the negotiation sails, not just on the question of the TRIPS waiver, but more broadly on all aspects of the trade negotiations going on at the WTO.

However, the onset of the Omicron wave further strengthened the logical case for a TRIPS waiver, even as the opponents continued to latch on to their arguments on intellectual property, driven largely by commercial considerations. On the one hand, the world was suffering on account of vaccine shortages, leading to faster and potentially deadlier mutations of the virus. On the other hand, the opponents of the waiver were worried about setting a precedent that they feared would get used more frequently if other crises were to hit the world.

Those in need wanted a solution today and those with the power to block continued to be worried about precedents of tomorrow, ignoring the devastation of today.

In recent years, the WTO has been coming under serious questioning on its relevance and effectiveness. The Director General of the WTO, Ngozi Okonjo-Iweala, personally took cognizance of this rapidly depleting trust of members to come up with a workable solution on the vaccine trilemma.

Starting mid-December 2021, Okonjo-Iweala, a seasoned Nigerian politician and erstwhile World Bank official, took initiative in convening a small group of just four members. The political leaders—ministers of trade, commerce and industry—of India, South Africa, the US and EU came together to start discussing a solution that would deliver the Covid-19 vaccines to the world at large.

This small group, dubbed Quad—yet another grouping of four members, started to meet regularly. Ministers Piyush Goyal of India, Ebrahim Patel of South Africa, Katherine Tai of the US and Valdis Dombrovskis of the EU got together with the leadership from the WTO in facilitating the meetings. These meetings would typically start after working hours in Geneva, also to accommodate the morning slots in the US. For India, this meant a midnight starting time, and the meetings continued late into the night; sometimes past 2.30 a.m. Goyal continued to put forth India's case strongly, without disturbing his normal routine of managing three large ministries and leading the upper house of the Parliament.

Hectic discussions ensued for almost three months in an effort to arrive at a solution backed by the key actors. The idea was that once the key actors agreed to a proposal, other members could be rallied around to accept the same under the masthead of the WTO.

On 15 March 2022, STAT, a website focussing on exclusive analysis of biotech, pharmaceutical and life sciences, leaked a draft proposal to which the small group of four members had apparently agreed. Though neither of the four governments made any official statement, Ed Silverman of STAT reported, 'After 18 months of talks, a compromise was reached on a proposal to waive intellectual property rights for Covid-19 medical products, according to a document shared with STAT and confirmed by a trade official familiar with the negotiations.'[57]

A tweet from the official Twitter handle of the WTO on 16 March further hinted that such a compromise had been reached.[58] The tweet was accompanied by a news report linking back to the media section of the website of the organization. It quoted Director General Ngozi Okonjo-Iweala, welcoming a breakthrough on the TRIPS waiver.[59]

The leaked text focussed on vaccines and not on diagnostics and therapeutics. This was different from the original submission made by India and South Africa. However, with the red lines drawn by developed countries that wanted to protect the commercial interests of their pharmaceutical companies, it was clear for a while that the intentions behind the 2 October 2020 proposal by India and South Africa had already been sabotaged.

The members of the WTO vociferously discussed and debated this text, dubbed as the Quad proposal, in the runup to the 12th

WTO Ministerial Conference in Geneva, which was held from 12 June to the early morning hours of 17 June in 2022. While the EU and US had negotiated within the four-member grouping with specific ideas, other members, like Norway, Switzerland and the UK, held on to their positions.

The outcome of the TRIPS waiver proposal hung in the balance through the 12th Ministerial Conference. Ultimately, in the wee hours of 17 June, the trade ministers agreed on the package of various deals. This included a decision on the TRIPS waiver, too—not the same proposal that India and South Africa had put forward in October 2020, yet an important win in the WTO, setting an important precedent on how to deal with global calamities.

Captured in the WTO documents WT/MIN(22)/30, also identified alternatively as WT/L/1141[60], the decision allowed interested members to use the flexibilities contained in the decision for five years. The decision also stated that the members would decide within six months on extending this decision to therapeutics and diagnostics areas, which were key to fighting the scourge of Covid-19.

The whole process of TRIPS waiver demonstrated how India fought a tough battle for the developing world, taking on entrenched global pharmaceutical lobbies as well as the developed world. With the initial support of South Africa and later bringing in a significant part of the WTO membership together, India led the battle for a global solution to the Covid-19 pandemic.

This battle ensured that India received a lot of goodwill from the developing world and from the Global South, which was generally deprived of the right quantities of the vaccine at the right moment. The proactive effort made by India in October 2020 ensured it a seat at the high table conducting global trade negotiations. This had never happened before. The fight also raised India's stature in global trade circles while also creating a template and a precedent to follow if the world were to face a similar situation again.

16

TAKING IT IN STRIDE

If there is one word that can summarize the myriad challenges faced by India through the pandemic, it would be 'scale'. As scale grows linearly, the complexity of the underlying system grows exponentially. Scale transformation is an underappreciated phenomenon in general, much less so when it comes to the problems of governance.

The pandemic management was a lesson in the effect of scale being an input to governance. What worked for a town would not necessarily work for another, even in the same state. What worked for a state would not hold any relevance for another.

The best demonstration of this phenomenon came early on in the onset of the pandemic. Through the first wave of Covid-19, global examples of pandemic management were unimaginatively thrown at India by the media and self-avowed intellectuals in the form of comparative studies. Cherry-picking of examples like New Zealand—a country with no land boundaries with any other neighbour, limited external connectivity and a population that would barely qualify to be the tenth-largest Indian city—and comparing its Covid-19 response to that of India, demonstrated the ignorance, or perhaps even malice, of those assuming the role of critics or specialists.

There was a lot of apprehension about India's state capacity to deliver a vaccination programme at all, let alone at the pace at which the programme eventually unfolded. There was some healthy scepticism, which was useful in shaping the public discourse towards potential impediments and focus on homegrown solutions. Then there was uninformed cynicism, where a section of the public intellectuals were absolutely sure India could never run an adult vaccination programme.

Finally, there was outright stereotyped dismissal—India, a poor, developing country cannot even think about nationwide vaccination. It was just not meant to be. Such a thought did not fit the colonial stereotypes, which dominate global media opinion on India. In this worldview, a 'regressive' India was always meant to be the recipient of wisdom being disseminated from the 'modern' West. Someone else always knew what was good for India, and the Indian job was to accept it at face value and merely implement the ideas.

There is an often an insistence that India should learn from global best practices. However, very little attention is paid to the assumptions, operating environment, social and economic conditions and nature of the institutions in which a particular best practice works. While a country should not be insular in formulating policies or course correcting existing ones, a simple lift and shift of a governance practice does not necessarily work equally effectively across countries without the underlying context demonstrating some similarities.

Ultimately, nothing succeeds like success, and this was very much the case with the Indian vaccination programme, too. The war with the real enemy—the virus—and the accompanying battles of perceptions and narratives were won through a national-scale indigenization. Understanding the pandemic in the Indian context, devising the solutions that would work locally, fine-tuning them to suit the vast and diverse expanse of the country and respecting the uniqueness of Indian circumstances is what won the day.

Aatmanirbhar Bharat has become a guiding light of sorts for India's governance and policy reforms after PM Modi exhorted the country to embrace the idea as the driving force behind Indian resurgence.[1] While India announced a series of reform measures after this address to the nation by the PM, aatmanirbharta, translated to self-reliance, ended up becoming a key pillar of the Indian vaccination programme.

Every aspect of the vaccination programme—India's development of the vaccine, diplomatic efforts to keep the supply chains open to get access to the components required for vaccine manufacturing, building trust in the vaccines so that almost universal coverage is achieved and resisting international pressures driven equally by omissions and commissions—required an indigenous assessment of the problem and a commensurate response.

While introducing the mantra of Aatmanirbhar Bharat to the country, PM Modi had remarked—'*Hamara sankalp is sankat se bhi virat hoga* (Our resolve will be much bigger than this problem).' Without an active demonstration and application of this national resolve, India would not have bounced back from the pandemic on its own terms.

Pressure to Buy mRNA Vaccines

A country with 1.37 billion people, each requiring two doses of a vaccine and perhaps a booster dose—what was a huge challenge for the Government of India was also a huge market opportunity for the pharmaceutical industry.

If every Indian was to be administered three doses of the vaccine—two in normal course and one as a booster, this was potentially a 4.5-billion-vaccine-dose market, accounting for some wastage and inventory handling problems. The mRNA vaccines were sold to the US at $19.5 per dose and to the EU at €15.5 per dose.[2] Smaller countries perhaps paid more.

Even if one assumes that these firms would have been 'benevolent' in their business offer to India and sold each dose at $20, India was a $90-billion market. This would not include the cost of the maintaining and running cold chains capable of handling these vaccines.

The Pfizer vaccine was initially designed to be transported and stored at -60°C to -86°C ultra-low temperature conditions.[3] India just did not have the required cold chains to make a public vaccination programme work under these operating conditions. The pharmaceutical firms did work on creating these conditions, but that happened much later in the vaccination journey.

At the time of the initial decision-making in the second quarter of 2020, the cold chain requirements themselves were far too onerous and impractical for India to adopt these mRNA vaccines. This problem was such a show-stopper that the prohibitive costs on top sounded like a distant second problem to deal with.

Then, there was the question of supply quantities. Would Pfizer and Moderna be able to actually commit to providing a significant number of vaccine doses in time for India? The vaccine supply situation was akin to the consumer goods shortages India used to face in 1970s and 1980s—there used to be a queue to buy a scooter or get a telephone connection. The monopoly supplier would enrol a willing participant in the queue and deliver based on its own supply constraints and opaque allocation algorithms.

Would it make sense for India to join a long queue, when the only prioritization option was to pay foreign suppliers an advance and hope that sovereign pulls and pressures did not impact the allocation algorithms? This would have been akin to leaving the national health policy in the hands of international pharmaceutical firms, who could decide the pace at and the direction in which the policy would move forward.

In fact, those queuing up and paying hefty advances also did not have a great experience[4] in terms of procurement and vaccine availability until the second quarter of 2021. Throwing money at a product constrained in supply and one that took its own path to a manufacturing ramp-up was always going to have its limits.

On top of the supply scarcity, Pfizer, in particular, had exigent contractual demands. Although there were no sovereign contracts signed in India with either Pfizer or Moderna, the analysis of these contracts appeared in the public domain over time. Some of the contractual arrangements sounded like treaty-backed neo-colonialism rather than a healthcare intervention.

First, there was no appetite for any bridging trial in India. The global pharmaceutical giants were reluctant to undertake any clinical trials to conform to Indian rules and regulations of approval. Even if that was to be accepted by the regulators, there was a derivative problem.

Second, these firms wanted contractual indemnity from any adverse events. As per a non-profit organization, Public Citizen, this required governments 'to indemnify, defend and hold harmless Pfizer' from and against any and all suits, claims, actions, demands, damages, costs and expenses related to vaccine intellectual property'.[5]

While it would not be unusual to have some immunity clauses in a contract like this, another non-profit, Transparency International, conducted an analysis of four contracts and concluded that the balance of the power was heavily in favour of the manufacturers and the national governments would have been on the back foot. It further observed that the contracts built 'more of the risk onto national governments, and away from the developer, even if missteps are made by the developer or supply chain partners, and not just if there is a rare adverse effect of the vaccines'.[6]

Third, the contracts provided Pfizer the ability to change critical terms and conditions, including dates of actual vaccine delivery itself, without any concomitant downside for the firm. This would have been too much of a risk for a public vaccination programme, in an environment of global competition for vaccines.

Fourth, Pfizer demanded public assets as collateral pledges to cover not just for any financial disputes but to also allow itself a fair amount of leeway to 'retaliate' should it consider a contracting government in breach of any clauses. As per the contracts with Brazil, Chile, Colombia, the Dominican Republic and Peru, which were analysed by various non-profits, governments were asked to 'expressly and irrevocably waive any right of immunity which either it or its assets may have or acquire in the future'.[7] Apparently some of these contracts also asked the governments to waive immunity against a precautionary seizure of their assets!

Fifth, Pfizer tried to control[8] even diplomatic engagements between sovereign nations and influence foreign policy by apparently controlling any donation mechanism within an intercountry arrangement.

Sixth, these contracts modelled private arbitration mechanisms in case of disputes and, hence, no national judicial proceedings could be initiated against the pharmaceutical firms.

Seventh, Pfizer even sought[9] to grant itself an intellectual property waiver while all along opposing the one being discussed in the WTO. Pfizer demanded that it be indemnified against any intellectual property claims against its vaccine or its components by the buyer.

Even then, the NEGVAC engaged in conversations with both Pfizer and Moderna throughout 2020. The signals from the pharmaceutical firms were lopsided—they would decide the quantities to be supplied, timing, pricing and, of course, use standard contractual terms, including the elements described above. Indian decision-makers were ill at ease with this attitude and language but continued to engage in discussions.[10]

The pressure from these firms, their domestic lobbyists and global amplifiers continued to mount in 2021. Especially after the second wave hit India badly, there were renewed attempts to influence public opinion. Public intellectuals, influential media voices and celebrities with no healthcare or governance exposure talked about Pfizer vaccines. There were innocuous-sounding tweets about people having taken the vaccine in a foreign country.

Opinion pieces and podcasts 'educated' people on why India was doing the wrong thing by not tapping into Pfizer. Whether these suggestions were made keeping in mind national interests or taken up expressly at the behest of the pharmaceutical firms in violation of Indian healthcare media regulations may never be known.

After the second wave, the NEGVAC restarted its discussion with Pfizer and Moderna to see if their vaccines could add to the national programme in any meaningful manner. Pfizer was willing to provide 50 million doses and Moderna just 7.5 million doses by the end of 2021.[11] These doses would be supplied at around $20 per dose and they, of course, came with the standard contractual terms, which would strangulate the government in case anything went wrong.[12]

These quantities were too small to make any difference to India's real requirements. Also, these vaccines would come so late in the year that their administration would not really make any significant additional impact in controlling the virus.

It was this small quantity on offer for which Indian authors, media personalities and entertainment business stalwarts put pressure on their own government to get Pfizer vaccines—clearly a targeted exercise.

For the sake of thoroughness, let us assume that India should have 'swallowed its pride' and done anything necessary to procure mRNA vaccines—pay the price, sign the indemnity clauses and everything else. After all, many richer countries did. And, of course, they placed their orders well ahead of time. Would that have ensured reliable supplies? In short, no. It wasn't physically possible at all. The reason can be summarized in two terms: 'air freight' and 'dry ice'. WHO guidelines[13] show that Pfizer/BioNTech vaccines must be kept at ultra-low temperature (ULT) of -60°C for long-term storage. Pfizer designed specialized transport boxes[14] for the purpose and only uses them for vaccine transport.

Each of these boxes weigh about 38 kg, most of it on account of the dry ice. A large refrigerated truck can hold about 60 such boxes, or about 3 lakh doses, weighing just over 2,200 kg. While a large aircraft can theoretically hold several truckloads worth—a Boeing 777-200F freighter has a revenue payload of over 1 lakh kg—the real payload capability is far lower. The reason is simple: federal aviation safety authorities restrict the maximum amount of dry ice a plane can carry. Originally just 3,000 lbs (1,360 kg), it was extended by the US Federal Aviation Administration to 15,000 lbs (6,800 kg) for Covid-19 vaccine transport, but this only applies to certain jurisdictions.[15] Excess dry ice in the hold can result in dry ice sublimation, overwhelming the aircraft's cabin pressurization.

As a result, the average transport flight for Pfizer vaccines between early to mid-2021 transported 2–5 lakh vaccines. Even this volume would require specialized ULT storage chains from the tarmac to hospitals, where a single ULT freezer costs upward of ₹25 lakh. The US and continental Europe were unaffected by these restrictions because they had local Pfizer/BioNTech production bases and vaccines could be transported anywhere in their geographic extent within days.

The alternative—sea freight—was out of the question, too. Pfizer's proprietary transport boxes are meant for a two-week transport duration. Ships from Europe to India take four to six weeks. There existed no ULT vaccine transport facility suited to those timelines, not to mention the fact that there wasn't enough production to supply the amounts India required. Transporting these vaccines to India and maintaining their operating conditions in the Indian ambience would have been very difficult if not outright impossible.

Health and Family Welfare Minister Mansukh Mandaviya assumed office in July 2021. While these discussions with the international pharmaceutical firms were going on, an Indian official of one of the firms paid him an introductory courtesy visit in the early days of his term.

Mandaviya was livid with this Indian official. He gave him

a piece of his mind on the usurious terms and conditions being imposed on India and that too for a very small number of vaccine doses relative to the Indian requirement. The minister did not even offer a chair to this particular visitor. Mandaviya was so enraged with the proposed documentation he had seen that he point-blank asked the Indian official whether it pinched his conscience to impose these terms on the country for the sake of corporate profits.[16]

All efforts of international lobbying and getting India to sign a bad deal were resisted by the government, keeping the national interests and priorities as the mainstay of decision-making. India's market was always going to be a big draw for the international pharmaceutical firms, many of whom made supernormal profits in the two years. However, India traversed this minefield with propriety without any negative impact on the vaccination programme itself.

Vaccine Hesitancy

Vaccine hesitancy was always going to be a big problem, which every country had accounted for. India was in the same boat with enough past experience of having handled this phenomenon in various other vaccine drives.

According to the WHO, 'Vaccine hesitancy refers to delay in acceptance or refusal of vaccination despite availability of vaccination services. The issue is complex and context specific, varying across time, place and vaccines. It is influenced by factors such as complacency, convenience and confidence.'[17]

The Ministry of Health and Family Welfare had released a detailed communication strategy to be used at central, state and district levels before the vaccination process began in India. This comprehensive document provided a detailed overview of the challenges the health authorities were likely to face. However, what transpired on the ground was very specific to local state and district contexts, and a lot of real time adjustments were required by the government machinery at various levels to ensure that people came forward to get vaccinated.

PM Modi took the lead in demonstrating that the vaccines were safe. Amidst early stage criticism about Covaxin and the approval process used by the Indian regulator, he showed to the country that the Made in India Covaxin was safe and he trusted the efficacy of the vaccine. His gesture was critical in building trust and removing the fear amongst people regarding vaccines.

At the same time, he waited for his turn based on CoWIN registration to get the vaccine and did not jump any queues. This also signalled to the country how the vaccination process would run. This discipline was followed in his office as well. When one of the co-authors of this book had scheduled the very first meeting with an official in the PMO to seek initial information, the meeting had to be postponed because the concerned official was queuing up with his family at a vaccination centre in New Delhi. Not using, let alone abusing, positional privileges became a feature of the process.

Such modelling is an important part of public communication. Voices that are considered relatable, inspirational or trustworthy help in addressing the anxiety about an uncertain health situation. This phenomenon was widely leveraged with a host of political leaders, movie stars, sports stars and public intellectuals talking about their vaccination experience. These known public figures shared pictures of themselves taking the vaccine on social media feeds, which became an important aspect of confidence-building process.

For the most part, the debate on vaccination in India did not fall prey to political squabbles and bickering. Barring a couple of exceptions, the Indian political establishment cutting across party lines expressed confidence in the vaccines. This was a critical difference from several countries, notably the US, where politicization of vaccine mandates hurt their eventual acceptance and uptake.[18]

Indian athletes, too, did not express any negative sentiments about the vaccines. This was a critical message because athletes are considered superhuman in their fitness regimes. If they were not worried about any adverse impact of vaccines, it was an encouragement for people at large to also not be worried.

While there were positive and trust-building stimuli at play with the help of public figures, the second wave of Covid-19 itself proved to be a fear stimulus. The fear it created goaded people to seek protection for themselves and their loved ones through the vaccine.[19]

The health authorities hit a series of localized problems. In Punjab, Covid-19 testing itself was hit badly as the farmers who were protesting against the liberalization of the Indian agriculture sector thought of Covid-19 testing as an excuse to break their protests and agitation. This hesitancy carried to vaccination, too. The local authorities had to patiently explain the benefits of not just the vaccination but the basics of the disease itself to turn the tide.[20]

In Dindori, Madhya Pradesh, a tribal district, local politicians had built up fear of the vaccine. In a district where health facilities were far from adequate, it was important that the residents did not shun the protection of the vaccines. However, there had been concerted campaigns against the vaccine by local politicians despite the fact that at the national level, politics had been left out of the vaccination debate. It took a lot of effort by the local Anganwadi workers and Accredited Social Health Activist (ASHA) workers to get people out of their houses for vaccination.[21]

In states like Chhattisgarh and parts of Madhya Pradesh, the ASHA workers and local public health centre workers became the target of social ostracization in some cases. Personal ties got strained because these workers were seen pushing the vaccination agenda. These local personal ties have, over the decades, proved to be very important to push better healthcare interventions. Such a disconnect between villages and community healthcare workers would not augur well, especially in states where maternal and infant health requires regular interfacing with these workers. These social costs of Covid-19 vaccination would take some time to reverse.[22]

In Mumbai, health researchers observed religion-based opposition to vaccination early on. This prompted local authorities to rope in religious leaders from the relevant communities to help build confidence regarding vaccines. This was not an easy process, as the imagined fear in this case was that the Covid-19 vaccinations reduced male fertility. This line of thinking was given credibility by individuals who sought to turn a scientific intervention into a social and political antagonism. However, the health authorities were able to eventually overcome this challenge.[23]

Similar challenges cropped up in different parts of the country. These were not linked to education or income levels. Overcoming these fears required dogged work. However, the fact that India did tide over these objections also shows how the country's primary healthcare infrastructure had matured over the years. While there is a long way to go on healthcare outcome improvements, the fact that public trust could be mobilized mainly through bottom-up action demonstrated the Indian fortitude in rising to the occasion.

Eventually, on 17 July 2022, India conquered the milestone of 2 billion doses. The efforts of vaccinators and the healthcare workers overcame both hesitancy and cynicism, sometimes at great personal cost to themselves. The sense of duty and selfless devotion that the healthcare workers brought to their job amply demonstrated that what India lacked in fiscal resources was more than made up by a humane touch.

No other large country could boast of having vaccinated more than 95 per cent of the eligible population once and more than 90 per cent adults twice.[24] The healthcare system overcame the pandemic and reinforced science through the values of personal accountability, empathy and humility. The WHO honoured[25]

India's over-1-million ASHA workers for furthering public health objectives at the seventy-fifth edition of its World Health Assembly in Geneva in May 2022.

Last Mile Access

As the vaccination programme ramped up through the third quarter of 2021, outperforming all expectations and demolishing all criticism, the focus shifted to two unique problems.

One issue that the government saw was that many individuals who had taken the first dose of the vaccine were skipping the second dose. This was perhaps an outcome of vaccine complacency, as the pandemic more or less subsided in India after June 2022. While there were local clusters of outbreak and rare cases of a sharp local increase in the case count, the virus seemed to have lost potency.

This had a reverse effect from the one observed after the second wave set in. Back then, the fear of the virus had made more people embrace the vaccine. But towards the fourth quarter of the year, the complacency and the misplaced belief that the virus was no longer a threat led to second doses being missed.

The second problem was that there were far-flung areas where it had not been possible to send vaccines and establish vaccination centres for a duration long enough to cover the entire population. Hamlets in hills, in deserts, on islands and in forests were still not fully saturated with vaccine coverage. Given that India had one of the highest vaccine acceptance rates, there was no reason not to reach out to the people living in these tough locales. But with the vaccine cold chain required to be maintained, this was not an easy task.

This is when India's community health spirit again came to the fore in awe-inspiring ways. The Ministry of Health and Family Welfare decided to get to each home in districts where the vaccine coverage had some gaps. On 3 November, the programme to knock on every door—*Har Ghar Dastak*—was launched by the ministry. The intent of the programme was creating further vaccine awareness and mobilization of resources for a specific objective, namely ensuring that the second dose was administered where due and the first dose coverage was increased. This programme was an exemplar of India's approach of 'no citizen being left behind' when it comes to the delivery of public services. With careful planning and unparalleled courage, magic started to happen.

In the Barmer[26] district of Rajasthan, a female health worker rode a camel, carrying vaccines in an ice-box to cross stretches of the Thar Desert and reached unvaccinated individuals.

In Dariyapur Saran village of Bihar, health workers had to walk through several streams and water bodies to reach the huts targeted for door-to-door vaccination. In Bihar,[27] remote access strategies like *Teeka Wali Naav* (boat with vaccines) and Motorbike Vaccine Team—vaccinators reaching distant areas on two-wheelers—were employed. A Refusal Response Team was constituted to convince the naysayers to accept vaccine doses.

In Budgam in Jammu and Kashmir, a severe cold wave in January 2022 did not dampen vaccinators' spirits. Wearing PPEs, female vaccinators walked long distances in the snow to reach[28] the elderly living in the upper reaches of the mountains and administered vaccines.

The story of Sangeeta Rawat[29] of Uttarakhand, an ASHA worker, inspired the country. Rawat would wake up early in the morning in Tapovan in the Chamoli district in Uttarakhand to undertake a 50-km one-way trip every day for several weeks. She would walk 7 km, undertaking an uphill climb, followed by a 43-km bus ride. Her travel to villages like Molta, situated at an altitude of 8,000 ft, would take six hours on way, often in sub-zero temperatures. It was the single-minded dedication of thousands of Sangeeta Rawats that carried the day for India.

No effort was spared in sending vaccines where they were needed. This included innovative use of technology, like drones.

Loukoipat, home to a beautiful ecological park on an island in Loktak Lake in Bishnupur, Manipur, got its supply of vaccines through special drone delivery planned by the ICMR.[30] The Drone Resource and Outreach in North East (i-DRONE) programme[31] had worked on such delivery vehicles, which could reach far-flung areas.

A similar initiative was also run in Karnataka. A CSIR drone was developed by the National Aerospace Laboratory and dubbed 'octacopter' in the Haragadde village in Anekal. This initiative helped in saving time taken for vaccine deliveries.[32]

The *Har Ghar Dastak* campaign also utilized locally relevant and innovative mobilization mechanisms.[33] The aim was to influence those who were still sceptical. Bihar ran a campaign *Ek Adhoora, Do Se Poora* (One is incomplete, two completes it), alluding to the importance of the second dose of the vaccine. Himachal Pradesh carried a message, '*Suraksha ke rang na honge pheeke, jab samay par lagenge do teeke.*' This literally translated to 'Safety will not wane when two vaccine doses will be administered on time.'

Awareness was also created through social events,[34] like *Kala Jathara*—troupes performing on traditional folklore in Andhra Pradesh and street plays in Jharkhand. These approaches used the blending of locally recognized means of mass communication with the message of vaccination acceptance.

The story of Raigarh in Chhattisgarh was unique. It was one of the earliest districts in India to achieve 100 per cent vaccine coverage in November 2021.[35] National Cadet Corps, National Service Scheme and Nehru Yuva Kendra Sangathan approached with hyperlocal mobilization strategies, including communication in local languages and dialects with a population that had a big tribal component and significant community engagement through existing networks—these formed the key in result orientation. Raigarh's success in running a complex vaccination campaign bottom-up, hamlet by hamlet, showed that the learning from

Indian democratic systems and processes, like elections, could be repurposed for public health programmes.

These examples demonstrate the efforts that went in the planning and execution of the vaccination programme. The *Har Ghar Dastak* programme played a key role in pushing vaccination coverage and ensuring that any potential regional and social inequities were successfully overcome with a proactive outreach.[36]

Cold Chain Adaptation

As India's process flow for vaccine movement got finalized in January 2021, the vaccine makers, like the SII and Bharat Biotech, were required to deliver the vaccines at regional centres in different states. These centres could be those run by the central government or by the respective state governments. From these centres, the appropriate government agency would then move the vaccines to their district warehouses and onwards to the vaccination centres.

Since private hospitals were also involved in the vaccination process after the initial few weeks, the vaccine makers also had to ship vaccines directly to the hospitals involved. This required the vaccine makers to partner with experienced cold chain operators, who could move vaccines over long distances.

The original points were Pune and Hyderabad, two cities that had bulk of the vaccine manufacturing capacities in place. From these two cities, trucks would be loaded and sent to different locations. In some cases, the vaccines were also shipped to the local airports and then carried by air routes to their destination. In this case, a cold chain arrangement was also required at the destination airport, so that the cargo hold area could receive and store vaccines until they were further loaded on to the delivery trucks.

One of the companies that became instrumental in this process, working with all Indian vaccine makers, was Kool-ex.[37] Based in Mumbai and Pune and run by entrepreneur Kunal

Agarwal along with his brother, Kool-ex has been operating in the pharmaceutical industry for more than a decade. The company had worked with these vaccine makers in other scenarios, so they found it easy to adapt their infrastructure to Covid-19 vaccines.

Vaccine transportation is a complex and technology-savvy exercise. The transportation assets are both top-quality construction and technology enabled. The structure of the truck, the reefer containers and the individual boxes carrying the vaccine are all built specifically for such a cold chain operation.

There are a lot of sensors inside the truck to understand if there are any events that may adversely impact the storage condition of the vaccines, including any temperature variations. Even for simple actions, like unauthorized truck opening, there are sensors mounted. The truck interior also has multiple sensors to understand the temperature profile while in transit. These sensors can be remotely monitored when the vehicles are in transit to understand variations in operating conditions. The vehicles themselves are enabled with GPS to track the location and movement on a real-time basis.

This was the kind of infrastructure deployed by Kool-ex for all movements of vaccines. Supply chains are the invisible heroes of any successful logistics-heavy business, but they are seldom recognized for their resilience. However, this was yet another area in which India's homegrown technology-led abilities carried the day perfectly, without any glitches or large-scale vaccine wastage.

While the manufacturers used Kool-ex to deliver the vaccines to the central or state government facilities, these still had to be moved further down to the next level—to districts and then to the vaccination centres. Some states used the services of Kool-ex for mid- and last-mile operations, too. But not all states could do so, given the general resource crunch. However, the vaccine manufacturers had ensured a very high-quality vaccine packaging, so that even without a Kool-ex-like service, states were able to keep the vaccines in play for the typical two-day window in which they were to be consumed.

In the first shipment of vaccines to kick-start India's public vaccination programme, Kool-ex transported 1.1 crore or 11 million vaccines in just 30 hours to various parts of the country from Pune.[38]

There were also very specific situations to be handled. When Sputnik V first arrived in India, the pre-manufactured doses had to be transported from the Hyderabad airport to the warehouses of the local partner, Dr. Reddy's Laboratories. Sputnik V required a temperature of -20°C for transportation. In this case, Kool-ex had to put their trucks in a pre-chilling mode five hours before the flight carrying the vaccines from Moscow landed in Hyderabad.

Kunal Agarwal personally waited for the flight to land at 3.00 a.m. to oversee the airport operation.[39] This was a different situation than carrying other vaccines. However, the Hyderabad airport had created arrangements for quick unloading, fast customs clearance and then truck loading of the vaccines in anticipation of the big event. The local police worked with Kool-ex to give a full route escort from the airport to the facilities of Dr. Reddy's Laboratories. A distance that may have taken two hours to traverse was covered in just 30 minutes with the help of local authorities.

The Pune airport has limited cargo handling capacities, as it is a space-constrained airport owned and managed by the IAF that also serves civilian operations. Two airlines—Air India and SpiceJet—started ferrying vaccines from Pune right from the beginning in January 2021, working with Kool-ex, despite the airports' physical limitations. By the end of the year, the Pune airport itself had handled more than 69 crore or 690 million doses of the vaccines.[40]

In general, Kool-ex had a very positive experience working with various central and state government agencies. The trucks carrying vaccines got priority movement in many cases. The state border clearances were without any glitches. In fact, on many occasions, the Kool-ex truck drivers reported that police escort vans used to wait for them to cross state borders and then guide them through to the final destination.

Kunal Agarwal reminisced about one such story. One of the earliest consignments from Pune had been shipped to Belgaum in Karnataka. This was the first consignment of vaccines reaching Belgaum and was eagerly awaited. The truck reached at 3.00 a.m. Even then, the recipient centre had arranged for a pooja of the trucks and the vaccine boxes. Men and women, dressed in elaborate traditional attire, accepted the vaccines with detailed rituals and with no less devotion than they would have demonstrated while praying in a temple. Sweets were distributed. One individual touched the feet of the truck driver, remarking that he was like Lord Hanuman carrying the famed *sanjeevani booti*.

Although the trucks carried prized and high-priced inventory, there were no instances of trucks being subjected to theft or hijack—events that are not uncommon in parts of the country that see regular cargo movement. In fact, in many states, people lined up on the roadsides to shower flower petals on the vaccine-carrying trucks. The truck drivers themselves had a very positive experience of interacting with the district and state authorities.

When the private hospitals entered the vaccination ecosystem, the work for companies like Kool-ex exploded. They were required to ship vaccines directly to the participating hospitals located in various parts of the country. At the peak of the vaccine movement, Kool-ex was covering about 20 lakh km or 2 million km of distance every month. This was akin to doing a round trip from the Earth to the moon three times in a month.

Yet again, Indian solutions worked for Indian conditions. A homegrown firm was able to undertake the entire national logistics operation, coordinating with the central government, state agencies and multiple vaccine manufacturers without any roadblocks or operational issues.

This significant environment of collaboration was yet another illustration of how Indian authorities, entrepreneurs and society rose to the occasion to exceed all expectations.

Diplomacy Keeping the Lights On in Factories

Export restrictions have been used as legitimate policy tools by countries in different emergency situations to take care of their national interests. This is understandable, because every country wants to protect its citizens first before helping others when a catastrophe hits. When it came to vaccine manufacturing, however, export restrictions led to some awkward situations. In fact, some became so grave that they actually threatened the viability of vaccine manufacturing itself.

The US invoked the Defense Production Act in March 2021,[41] which prevented the American firms from exporting any and all components of vaccines, not just the finished vaccines themselves. The Defense Production Act had originally come into force in September 1950 in the aftermath of the Korean War. It enabled the President of the US and American federal agencies to influence the domestic industry to act in a way that aligned with the national interest. Although it was meant to be a war-time emergency mechanism, the Act, effective since 1950, has been invoked more than 50 times.[42]

In relation to the Covid-19 vaccines, invocation of this Act severely hampered the ability of vaccine makers in India to access critical raw material. The US was a key manufacturer and exporter of basic vaccine ingredients and manufacturing equipment, and its export ban led to an immediate global shortage. Vaccine makers could not access items like reagents, nano-filters, tubing and specialized disposable bags, all of which were required to make any vaccine.[43]

The global shortage was caused by the technicality of the American laws. Suppliers, like Cytiva and Pall Corporation and Thermo Fisher, were obliged by law to fulfil the needs of American vaccine makers and pharmaceutical companies first. Only when that demand was fulfilled could they honour the contracts signed overseas. But the demand of American vaccine makers and pharmaceutical firms for these components was limitless, just like other global firms in the business.

The SII took a hit in the production of Covishield as well as Novavax production. It could not source even basic raw material like the specific medium needed to grow microorganisms on account of this export ban by the US.[44]

Bharat Biotech had another problem. It had signed a deal in October 2020 with Kansas-based biotechnology company ViroVax, founded by researcher Sunil David.[45] ViroVax would provide Bharat Biotech with the adjuvant Algel-IMDG, a pharmacological agent used to boost immune response of a vaccine.[46] Although this adjuvant had not been used before in any vaccine, Bharat Biotech had conducted extensive trials using this unique ingredient and the vaccine had worked well. The American policy threatened the potential supply of the adjuvant, without which Covaxin could not be produced.

India took up these concerns with the US formally and strongly.[47] As the infections climbed through April and May 2021, External Affairs Minister Dr S. Jaishankar spoke to his American counterpart, Secretary of State Antony Blinken, on 19 April. In a conversation that focussed on the close cooperation India and the US enjoyed in several spheres, including international affairs, Jaishankar stressed on the importance of ensuring that Indian vaccine makers did not face problems.

This conversation was then followed up by India's Ambassador to the US, Taranjeet Sandhu, who kept approaching American officials in Washington DC. The Indian embassy also got regular feedback from the Indian manufacturers of the actual issues on the ground so that solutions could be devised and facilitated.

After several rounds of discussions and application of deft democracy, Indian vaccine manufacturers got the good news on

3 June 2021. The Biden administration in the US decided to remove[48] the Defense Production Act ratings on AstraZeneca, Novavax, Sanofi vaccines, leading to a sigh of relief at both ends of the Deccan plateau in India.

Indian diplomacy played a big role in nudging the US to review and change its policy, which lasted three months. During these three months, the negotiations on the intellectual property waiver on Covid-19 vaccines and other relevant goods had also intensified in the WTO in Geneva.

The Biden administration had itself indicated support for a potential intellectual property waiver with a willingness to enter the negotiations. This prodding from different directions eventually helped Indian firms to get the outcome they sought. The SII chief Adar Poonawalla formally thanked[49] Jaishankar and Indian diplomatic efforts on this front.

In an interesting turn of events, the US itself fell back on the production of vaccines in 2022. Both Pfizer and Moderna took the production of their highly sought-after vaccines to Europe, perhaps fearing that the US policies may disrupt their commercial interest. The invocation of the Defense Production Act was cited[50] as a key reason by the American think-tanks for this change of fortune of the American pharmaceutical industry.

International Vaccine Recognition and Approvals

'Proof of vaccination' became an international requirement to travel. Almost every country introduced what came to be dubbed as 'vaccine passports'—needed to arrive in or transit via a country.

Different countries used their definition of what was 'fully vaccinated' and allowed only those individuals to travel freely who had taken the recognized vaccines. Others had to undertake a Covid-19 test to travel, often leading to additional testing costs, administrative overhead and travel chaos.

Unfortunately, this process became a geopolitical tool in itself.

Several countries took their time in recognizing Covaxin as one of the accepted vaccines. This inconvenienced many Indians who had to change or delay their travel plans to deal with the complex entry requirements imposed by the countries they intended to travel to. One of the reasons for this situation was the delay in Covaxin getting WHO approval and recognition.

While the WHO recognized several vaccines, it took almost 10 months for Covaxin to make the cut after getting an EUA in India. It was only on 3 November 2021 that Covaxin got the coveted listing, becoming the eighth vaccine globally to be listed.[51] It appears that there were challenges on both sides leading to this delay.

Bharat Biotech has been a scientist-led operation, with Dr Krishna Ella personally focussing on the research and intellectual property aspects. Unlike other pharmaceutical giants from the West, who invest heavily in managing governmental and inter-governmental relations, Bharat Biotech has been focussed on the core business.

The company could have potentially kept the global health authority in the loop during its clinical trial process. But this communication was not prioritized over the regular research, clinical trial, production and distribution functions, which were critical to get the vaccine to the market. On the other hand, the WHO did issue emergency listing for other vaccines, where there is no evidence that similar scrutiny had been conducted as was done for Covaxin.

Irrespective of what transpired, the Indian public at large was left with the impression that there was a bias regarding the country of origin when it came to the emergency listing process. The widespread belief in India has been that some vaccines were potentially privileged over others and the reasons for the same may not have been purely scientific or medical in nature.

Worse still, even after the Covaxin emergency listing, several countries continued to impose restrictions on movement of those who had taken the vaccine. India also, in turn, continued to adjust reciprocal privileges, maintaining diplomatic pressure to ease the situation.

A bizarre situation arose when, in September 2021, the UK omitted Covishield from its list of vaccines, which allowed travellers to access the country without additional restrictions. Covishield was just the Indian version of a British vaccine, so this move could not have been vaccine efficacy related. Later, the UK clarified that its concern was about the incompatibility of the vaccine certificates issued through CoWIN and those by its National Health Service.[52]

India also imposed reciprocal quarantine restrictions on the individuals travelling from the UK to India until this situation got resolved. It took about a month to bring this episode to an amicable conclusion. But it showed how the pandemic led to protectionism, which often targeted Indian interests.

When one of the co-authors of this book met PM Modi in his office in New Delhi on 16 July 2021 in a conversation unrelated to this book, he asked the PM how he deals with the pressure of the job.[53] PM Modi remarked, 'A person who is not weak does not get angry about problems. Instead he uses the pressure to bring out the best.' That spirit clearly drove the vaccination journey, wherein every day brought new challenges for the government, not just on account of the pandemic but also motivated pressure to steer their decisions in particular directions.

Ultimately, these unique situations that Indian policymakers addressed through the course of the pandemic could only be possible due to a whole-of-government approach. The severity of the problems motivated the country to do more. The numerous battles that were fought and more often than not won helped the country win the bigger war. What the country learnt in the journey is already in the process of being institutionalized.

17

LEADERSHIP: DOING THE RIGHT THINGS

The phrase 'once-in-a-lifetime pandemic' was liberally used in the early days of the Covid-19 outbreak. The confidence in that phrase seems to have evaporated since, with an air or general resignation that such an event may indeed occur again in one's own lifetime.

One of the key characteristics of political leadership is to steer the country in the right direction. National leaders not just determine what needs to be done but also show the path to accomplish these goals and overcome challenges. Doing the right things defines effective leadership.

This is the key message the Indian establishment has taken from the pandemic. As uncertainty and ambiguity became the calling cards of a transitional world, PM Modi guided a series of steps that sought to institutionalize the learnings from the pandemic-handling experience, especially with respect to the vaccination process.

The changes that need to be brought in are structural in nature, which, when implemented fully, will produce a more effective response to any equivalent future health crisis. While it is tempting to solve the problem when it arises—and it is, of course, important that this is done by the governance machinery—what is often more important and critical is to manage the genesis of the problem itself.

Can a crisis be averted altogether? If not, can its onset be delayed? Can its impact on the population be reduced once it is in play? Can the country bounce back faster from the crisis? These questions require long-term and institutional solutions, over and above the ability to respond to a problem that stares the country in the face.

As the Covid-19 pandemic demonstrated, health crises may often be exogenous. Hence, it may also be tougher to model or predict them, given the very broad range of factors that may contribute to precipitating such crises. The national infrastructure should, hence, be ready to deploy all strategies in the arsenal—avoid, delay, react, respond, limit, spring from—to deal with emerging situations. This is the approach the government sought to take through its policy responses once the immediate task of protecting the country through the vaccines had been achieved.

Breaking Silos

One of the traditional criticisms of the Indian governance setup has been a silo mentality, where different ministries, departments or institutions may not always work together very efficiently. These entities may be very good at implementing their own agenda but often don't come together to form the bigger picture.

When PM Modi assumed office in May 2014, he started work on dismantling this silo mentality in the administration.[1] He encouraged officials from different ministries to work together to formulate end-to-end solutions to problems rather than working with the spirit of limited local optimization.

Over the years, this change has reflected in various ways in the conduct of the government. Be it the initiatives like PRAGATI, which the PM undertakes to review the progress of signature infrastructure projects, formation of the GST Council in the spirit of federalism or new programmes like PM Gati Shakti, aimed at bringing cross-functional solution orientation to common problems, the idea has been to break silos.

Hence, when the National Task Force on Covid-19 was

announced on 18 March 2020, various parts of the government spread across ministries and departments came together seamlessly to address the problem at hand. This task force, hosted under the chairpersonship of Dr V.K. Paul of the NITI Aayog, ensured that the Indian Covid-19 response was cross-functional, granular and well coordinated.

This National Task Force, and later the NEGVAC, which also had specific responsibilities assigned to different organizations and individuals, played a key role in not just making quick decisions, but also in ensuring that the decisions were implemented.[3] Without such an institutional arrangement, the Indian response, specifically the local development of vaccines, may not have been so effective.

The NEGVAC met very frequently, discussing all aspects of the vaccination challenge openly and clearly. While each subgroup was working on its own tasks, the regular coordination ensured that every individual and organization was aware of the problems to overcome. They were able to closely collaborate whenever such a need arose. This decision by PM Modi to bring a whole-of-government approach to the Covid-19 management became the defining pillar of the Indian response.[4]

The agility of decision-making in the Covid-19 management as well as in the national vaccination programme also emanated from the fact that there was a political backing for the administrative machinery. The officials across ministries were able to work together and bring new ideas to execution quickly because the government acted as a willing and staunch backstop.

This approach is a good template for any future such situations, that would require multiple ministries to coordinate to solve a national problem and define structural solutions. Process reforms are an integral part of how governance evolves, and the template drawn by PM Modi is a milestone in such reforms.

Pradhan Mantri Ayushman Bharat Health Infrastructure Mission

PM Modi launched the Ayushman Bharat Health Infrastructure Mission in Varanasi on 25 October 2021. Speaking at the launch of this mission to transform healthcare infrastructure, the PM said, '[...] Shiva and Shakti reside in Kashi. Kashi, the powerhouse of knowledge, relieves us from both pain and suffering. Then what better place than Kashi to start such a mega plan related to health and such a huge resolution to get rid of diseases and sufferings?'[5]

This is the largest pan-India health infrastructure upgradation programme, which was announced by the Finance Minister Nirmala Sitharaman in her budget speech[6] on 1 February 2021 with an outlay of ₹64,180 crore or about $8.4 billion over six years.

The measures proposed under this scheme focus on developing capacities of health systems as well as preparing them in responding effectively to the current and future pandemics or other potential disasters.[7] The central government proposed to undertake this upgrade from its budget, though public health is largely a state subject in India.

A network of public health laboratories and infectious disease hospitals are proposed to be built across all the districts in the country. Creating local diagnosis capabilities would help in having a faster response to infectious diseases. Reflecting on the time when all Covid-19 test samples were shipped to Pune in the initial days of the outbreak, this ambition will be a huge positive change.

This network[8] will include facilities in 730 districts and 3,500 chosen rural blocks nationally. The government also plans to create an enabling framework of disease surveillance to be deployed in the densely populated metropolitan cities, where the chances of a spread of infectious diseases can be higher.

These investments also have knock-on effects on demand for healthcare professionals in addition to creating high-quality local jobs. This, in itself, will provide a boost to India's healthcare service delivery through a cycle of virtuous positive feedback loops. The number of seats that India today has for medical education as well as allied services, like nursing, are already being increased.

An important aspect of this funding is to create a network of Viral Diagnostic and Research Laboratories, including BSL-3 and 4 facilities across the country. During the development of Covaxin, the presence of a limited number of BSL-3 sites came to the fore. These are required to handle deadly pathogens and the process of their inactivation.

India also plans to establish the National Institute of One Health, regional centres for the National Centre for Disease Control and new National Institute of Virology through this central government programme.

Finally, this programme will enable a network of health emergency operation centres and localized initiatives, like mobile health facilities, for better response to future health crises.

National Institute of One Health

The government has taken up the concept of One Health expeditiously. A common consensus is emerging globally that zoonotic diseases may lead to future global health events. These diseases transmit across species from animals to humans or from humans to animals. Their greater prevalence and potential to impact public health means that the governments need to know more about them and the risks they pose.

India has taken cognizance of this situation. The One Health Consortium[9] comprising India's leading hospitals, medical research centres and universities has been established to study the prevalence of 10 selected zoonotic diseases, which may potentially spread across India. This consortium will also study five trans-boundary animal diseases, with a special focus on the northeastern states sharing land boundaries with other countries. The work of the consortium will help forewarn public health authorities of any future disease outbreaks.

The ICMR is in the initial stages[10] of establishing a dedicated centre in the form of National Institute of One Health. This will come up at Nagpur and will also house a BSL-4 laboratory. The vision for this institute is to work on the idea of 'One Health' involving cross-functional experts, including veterinarians, ecologists, wildlife experts, epidemiologists and public health experts. The centre also expects to collaborate with other research organizations, similar bodies in other countries and with the WHO.

Bringing together animal health, human health and environmental and ecological considerations may be the key to a significantly better pandemic response, and India will play a crucial role towards this objective.

Regional Institutes for Virology and BSL-3 Facilities

The Union Budget for the financial year 2021–22 outlined the plan to set up four new NIVs. The budget also provides for nine new BSL-3 facilities. These will help the government understand all pathogens of interest better and quicker.

When the Covid-19 virus surfaced, China, which has a network of multiple such facilities, was able to identify the virus and actually sequence the virus in a matter of just 10 days.[11] This type of capability is important to build, as national response may have to take precedence even though India works closely with international bodies.

The vulnerabilities of the global health architecture were exposed during the Covid-19 pandemic. These new facilities will help India tide over the concerns emanating from a lack of international information flow. These new institutes will also provide a fillip to local research capabilities in epidemiology and beyond.

The NIV, Pune, established in 1952, will also get some well-deserved support after seven decades. The Pune institute has been instrumental in enhancing the country's understanding about pathogens and devising strategies. It also has ample experience in supporting these greenfield facilities.

Technology Repurposing

The CoWIN platform stood the test of scale, speed and complexity, setting a very high bar of what a public health technology intervention will look like.

The government now plans to extend[12] the use of CoWIN in the UIP. Given the smaller volumes handled in the vaccination programme, which is aimed at covering expecting mothers and newborns, the scale of the intervention will be significantly lower than a national adult vaccination programme.

Bringing the UIP on CoWIN will digitize the entire vaccination process, making it easier for the health workers to track and follow up on this critical public health intervention. This also takes away the need for physical vaccine certificates and tracking documents. The CoWIN platform can generate vaccination certificates, which can be stored digitally[13] in a system like DigiLocker, which is quite popular already as a cloud storage public digital asset.

India's UIP covers[14] inoculation for 12 diseases, all preventable by the use of vaccines. These include polio, diphtheria, tetanus, measles and hepatitis B, among others. The vaccine shots are administered by the government free of cost.

Another key advantage of using CoWIN for the UIP is that the rolled-up aggregate data will become a big source of health analytics. This will also spur evidence-based policymaking on health interventions, including understanding regional trends, right up to the village level.

The application may also be a useful intervention for any healthcare 'supply–demand matching' processes such as organ donations and blood bank management. These ideas are also being explored.[15]

Confidence in Indigenous Ideas and Solutions

The management of Covid-19 pandemic highlighted the need to design and develop local solutions and, more importantly, trust that these work. There is a natural tendency to agree with what comes from global agencies or 'foreign intellectuals'.

This became very evident in how the parameters of the SARS-CoV-2 were defined and how prescriptions were handed from global health authorities. Their credibility may not have been in question, but the frenzy generated by their prescriptions and the pressure built on sovereign states to accept the 'do as I say' approach left an unpalatable sentiment.

It almost appeared that the technocracies around the world were seeking to establish some kind of global government, with no legitimacy to dictate to governments but significant clout in the name of science. The narrative monopolies in the media and academic industry then drummed up the commands of these technocracies and unleashed campaigns of shaming anyone who had even a mildly different position on any aspect of how the virus behaved.

Is SARS-CoV-2 airborne? This question was asked[16] by Shekhar C. Mande, then director general of the CSIR in a blog[17] written on his organization's website in July 2020. The CSIR even worked on formal studies[18] exploring such possibilities.

However, the western health regulators and global health authorities had been invested in the idea of droplet-based transmission. In the initial months, all studies were focussed on this concept, including exploration of potential mitigation actions. It took the WHO almost two years to accept that the virus was airborne[19] and, hence, issues like ventilation and indoor crowding were of consequence.

Indian Covid-19 treatment protocol always maintained the importance of ventilation, and it was reinforced[20] as the infections progressed. Based on the work done by the CSIR, India adopted specific detailed building management procedures released by NITI Aayog.[21]

Based on the recommendations of the CSIR, India also issued guidelines for and started the process of installation of ultraviolet air sanitizing solutions. This process was undertaken[22] in the Indian Parliament, along with public spaces, like buses and trains.

Although not directly linked to vaccination, this example underscores how indigenous ideas not only proved to be correct, but, in fact, were ahead of the time in terms of how the global view on the pandemic evolved. This approach will likely reflect more in policymaking in the future.

Global Vaccine Partnerships

Through the course of the pandemic, it was clear that the vaccine trilemma—access, equity and affordability—was not going to be easy for any country to meet. Barring the countries that had the combination of financial muscle and domestic access to vaccines—both being necessary conditions—every other country or blocs of countries faced problems with at least one of the three dimensions.

While India conducted swift and engaging bilateral vaccine diplomacy, the country also looked at institutional mechanisms for global vaccine partnerships in addition. The Quad Vaccine Partnership, part of the Australia, Japan, India and US grouping dubbed Quad, pledged to donate 1.2 billion doses of vaccines in the Indo-Pacific region.[23] The four Quad members realized that global initiatives were important in targeted delivery of vaccines, solving the country-specific dimensions of the trilemma.

These Quad vaccines were largely produced by the Indian firm Biological E. The process of handing over these vaccines to the countries in Indo-Pacific region started with Thailand.[24]

The Quad leaders' declarations were focussed on Covid-19. But the text[25] indicates that the thinking may be easily reused and some elements of the current plan, like the 'global pandemic radar' and improvements to viral genomic surveillance may have applicability beyond Covid-19, too.

In keeping with PM Modi's regular exhortation of the sentiment of *Vasudhaiva Kutumbakam*, India is in a position to use its manufacturing prowess and supply chain resilience for predictable access to pandemic goods.

The former President of the US, John F. Kennedy, once remarked: 'When written in Chinese, the word "crisis" is composed of two characters—one represents danger and one represents opportunity.'[26] It is not clear if Kennedy got his etymology right, but the spirit of his articulation was spot on.

There is no better example of how this spirit reflected in India's vaccination programme. The programme turned a crisis into a manageable tragedy, one that inflicted huge losses but could not obliterate the collective resolve of the country.

Valuable lessons have been learnt for the future, none more important than focussing on building an Aatmanirbhar Bharat.

18

AATMANIRBHAR BHARAT

Since PM Narendra Modi spoke about Aatmanirbhar Bharat for the first time in May 2020, there has been a vibrant debate in the country on what really is the meaning of aatmanirbharta.

A simple English translation would mean self-sufficiency. Taking this literal interpretation, there has been a criticism of the concept of Aatmanirbhar Bharat, as those who hold the ideals of globalization dear see this from a narrow lens of economic self-sufficiency. Narrowing down this fear further, the critics equate Aatmanirbhar Bharat with the tried, tested and failed ideas of self-sufficiency so popular in the Indian socialist narrative.

The popular argument goes that no country in the world can truly be self-sufficient. One has to play by international rules to ensure that symbiotic relationships between countries are shaped by mutual economic dependence. That economists think of economics, trade, open borders and interdependence as the grease that reduces international friction is hardly surprising.

The world has, however, taken a turn for greater complexity and considerations beyond economics. Technocrats around the world, who tend to be stateless globalists in their thinking and writing and nativist in the glorification of their own ideas, have for most part missed this trend. An obvious reason may be that a less integrated world hurts the core economics and personal interests of those who benefit from such integration.

Elected politicians in every country, however, have to look beyond these idiosyncratic dogmas because, unlike the technocrats, they are actually accountable to people of their respective countries. Ideas may be global, but their impact—positive or negative—is felt differently in different countries, playing out in the proximate context. The pandemic has exposed precisely these unequal fissures and tensions, punctuating commonly accepted socio-economic theories with harsh real-world costs to lives and livelihoods.

The unwinding of globalization was already on with the distributional inequalities of trade and development causing intra-as well as inter-country conflicts. But major geopolitical shifts cannot be modelled in oversimplified binaries. Unwinding or decoupling does not mean disconnection.

The pandemic brought home the reality that if greater global integration benefitted through economics, the receding of the same integration accentuated social problems in an even bigger way. Economic integration was unable to build lasting trust in the global order, where the bullwhip effect of some bats flying in Wuhan led to the world getting rewired.

The pandemic has exposed the underbelly of a world where anything and everything that promotes convergence can also be weaponized to engineer rapid and serious divergence.

Corporate balance sheets, financial muscle, food grains, intellectual firepower, manufacturing prowess, media, multilateral institutions, science journals, social media and technology are all purveyors of a world that has been coming closer, both in terms of flow of ideas as well as flow of resources. However, each of these levers of globalization, with absolutely no exception, has also been weaponized during or in the aftermath of the pandemic.

The tail event—where many of these elements are used concurrently and simultaneously by those who control them—can be really difficult for any country to navigate. It is this tail event that the idea of Aatmanirbhar Bharat seeks to address.

What Self-Sufficiency Really Means

Each country has to identify what levers of globalization can be short circuited and by whom to bring its journey in the international order to an abrupt halt. An Aatmanirbhar Bharat will ensure that when the external dependencies don't work, when there are exogenous shocks and when those expected to help India have gone into a shell—to look for their own or to act against Indian interests—India still keeps running on the path of development.

Vaccines led this idea by example. Had the first pit stop for Aatmanirbhar Bharat been another commodity that already existed and where the know-how was easily available, perhaps the depth of the idea may not have been appreciated. But because vaccines were needed here and now, and India did not have existing intellectual property in this specific area of vaccines, the success hit hard in a good way.

The vaccination programme depended on two Indian strengths—scaling up an available knowledge base, and quick and relatively less costly innovation using ideas with greater probability of success. That these strengths delivered in the present convinced us that Aatmanirbhar Bharat was not a slogan. If India could do this in the face of the biggest global calamity since the Second World War, it could also replicate the favourable outcome without the proverbial gun to the head.

In this sense, Aatmanirbhar Bharat allows us a chance to step back and survey what aspects of our lives we need to do well in to keep the society and the country insulated from external shocks. In fact, this survey and analysis may well lead to a conclusion that we need to integrate more with certain parts of the world. But such a conclusion will be drawn based on our understanding of the emerging geopolitics. India will act with a balance of beliefs, values and interests in mind, but most importantly the balance will be decided through our own understanding of the global order.[1]

The idea of Aatmanirbhar Bharat also appreciates and recognizes the unique circumstances of the Indian nation. A country with more than one-sixth of the world's population and just over $2,000 per capita income has to devise strategies that work for it. Using the best practices and learning from the world is fine as long as the learning also leads to the understanding of what may not work. Aping other countries without appreciating their context has not really helped India in the past, and there is no reason why borrowed ideas may do any better in the future.

Thinking for Ourselves

Scale is the defining Indian feature that persuades policymakers to think for themselves. An Aatmanirbhar Bharat needs to start with an aatmanirbhar thought process, with space for empirical testing of what works and what does not. Throughout this book, a common theme has been that of execution at scale, accomplished under immense and continuous pressure, constrained by various factors within and outside the control of the government. This experience should give us the confidence that aatmanirbhar thinking works, and there should be no reason to not shed the hesitations of history.

Historically, Indian delivery systems have underachieved not just the potential but invariably also the explicit promise. This is perhaps a reason why there is an automatic scepticism about an Aatmanirbhar Bharat. This chronic delivery failure or long denial of basic public goods and services, like roads, electricity, water, sanitation and housing, may have germinated a question mark on bigger ambitions. However, the country has indeed changed discontinuously.

India now delivers not just what is required for a dignified day-to-day living but goes beyond linear extrapolations to achieve what much of the better-equipped world can't. Perhaps, there are gaps between the two extremes to fill, but the intent to fill these gaps is very much there. An Aatmanirbhar Bharat can only accelerate this process.

What happens in the coming decades is an exercise in crystal ball gazing, likely beyond the bounded rationality of any observer today. What matters, however, is to be prepared for whatever comes India's way, without getting fazed.

Addressing a programme titled '*Azadi Ke Amrit Mahotsav se Swarnim Bharat Ke Ore*', PM Modi urged:

> Amrit Kaal [the twenty five years from 2022 to 2047 leading up to 100 years of Indian independence] is not for dreaming while sleeping, but for fulfilling your resolutions awake. The coming 25 years are the period of utmost hard work, sacrifice, and 'tapasya'. This is a period of 25 years to get back what our society has lost in hundreds of years of slavery.[2]

Aatmanirbhar Bharat stands for this ambition and devotion to the cause. It does not imply that the country is running away from the world. It stands for an India that knows its strengths, an India that will work on honing these strengths and an India that will use these strengths unapologetically when required. The aatmanirbhar vaccination programme was just the first step and there is a long way to go.

This Aatmanirbhar Bharat will be capable and confident beyond the two poles of arrogance and diffidence.

PM Modi said in an address to the Indian community in Singapore in 2015, '*Na hum aankh jhuka kar baat karenge, na aankh dikhaa kar baat karenge. Hum duniya se aankh mila kar baat karenge* (We will talk to the world as equals, not from a position of superiority or inferiority).'[3]

May India prevail.

AFTERWORD

India has always been known as the 'Pharmacy of the World'. That was true even during the Covid-19 pandemic, where India was self-reliant in making enough vaccines. We were even able to supply many vaccines to other nations.

India showed the world that a country can overcome stiff challenges when its scientific minds and medical professionals come together with the right policy support from the government. India has never been short of ideas and ingenuity. When this spirit of exploration and risk-taking meets the right operating environment, India can do wonders.

Let us not forget for a minute that what we achieved on the vaccination front was nothing short of a wonder. A country with such a large population and with so many variations across states could still achieve more than 2 billion vaccine doses in a planned and organized manner. In hindsight, this may sound easy. But at the start of the pandemic, very few people would have given India a shot at such a staggeringly high quality of self-reliant execution.

We were able to get a USFDA approval for a new vaccine, which is a unique feat. No Indian company has ever achieved this feat in vaccines. This step opens the door for the industry, and no country can look at India as an inferior player.

It is a matter of immense happiness that this journey chronicling a true Indian accomplishment has been documented in Aashish Chandorkar and Suraj Sudhir's book *Braving a Viral Storm: India's Covid-19 Vaccine Story*. When the achievement is fresh in our minds, looking back on how the country came out of a dark storm is very satisfying.

Serum Institute of India (SII) had a 1.5-billion-dose capacity before the pandemic. Now we have an over 4-billion-dose capacity, which includes bulk manufacturing. That's thanks to the new global pandemic facility we have invested in, which can handle multiple technologies like messenger RNA (mRNA). So, all that infrastructure is now ready and is being commissioned.

Going forward, the vaccine industry and SII, in particular, will focus on innovation and developing new vaccines to treat diseases. For example, next year, for the first time in India, a Made in India human papillomavirus (HPV) vaccine to prevent cervical cancer in women will be launched.

Other Indian vaccine manufacturers have also invested in and built additional capacity. So, the total Indian capacity of vaccines may be around 7 to 8 billion doses. As the pandemic recedes, the available capacity can be deployed in the future as per the evolving requirements.

For an industry like vaccines to work, transparency and trust are very important. The government has done a wonderful job to achieve such vaccine coverage. We must highlight Prime Minister Narendra Modi's leadership. I am extremely optimistic regarding the environment and the policies that he has provided to the industry. With these, India will continue to be a global leader in this field.

Adar Poonawalla,
CEO and owner,
Serum Institute of India

ACKNOWLEDGEMENTS

Writing a book is incredibly exhilarating and nerve-wracking at the same time. It is a labour of love but also carries immense weight of expectations. Working on a book that addresses contemporary history and, in fact, events that are still playing out in front of us, is doubly daunting. One's hope should stay separate from one's analysis, lest a contradiction emerge as the readers hold the book in their hands.

This book would not have been possible without the inspiring leadership of Prime Minister Narendra Modi. His second term almost immediately ran into the biggest global crisis since the Second World War. His leadership and the ability to put India's interests first and foremost are qualities that are incredibly motivating. His office extended all the help required in piecing together this story and answering difficult questions.

Union Minister for Health and Family Welfare Mansukh Mandaviya detailed several nuances of India's spirited fight against the virus and the unreal challenges that we overcame. His office provided insightful information and data that was very helpful in writing the book.

The book would not have taken shape without the trust shown by Kapish Mehra and Yamini Chowdhury of Rupa Publications in this work. Their assistance and feedback were instrumental in shaping the book. Aurodeep Mukherjee and Sakschi Verma did a thorough job of reading and editing the manuscript. Many aspects of the research for the book were handled by Abhinav Joshi, a young public policy professional and Kuhuo Bajaj, a young student with immense love for the country. We are thankful to both.

The authors interviewed several individuals whose unique insights enriched the understanding of the authors as well as moulded the contents of the book. We are especially grateful to Adar Poonawalla, Amit Paranjape, Anand Ranganathan, Ashok Malik, Balram Bhargava, Hiren Joshi, Hitesh Jain, K. VijayRaghavan, Krishna Ella, Kunal Agrawal, Mona, Nimish Joshi, Nirav Shah, Oommen Kurian, Peter Hotez, Pratyasha Rath, Priyam Gandhi-Mody, Rahul Bajoria, Rajiv Nath, Ram Prasad, Ram Sewak Sharma, Raman Gangakhedkar, Randeep Guleria, Sanjay Singh, Sanjeev Sanyal, Sanjeev Navangul, Satish Mehta, Shekhar Mande, Vivek Agnihotri, V.K. Paul and Vaibhav Bajaj for their help. The one thread that bound us with them was the keenness to put forward the incredible story of India's achievements and the desire to see India succeed.

Several senior officials from the Indian government across ministries and research institutions as well as those working in international organizations, like the World Health Organization, Gavi and World Trade Organization (WTO) in Geneva, helped in piecing together events and stories. These officials did not want to be named. The authors, however, are grateful for their contribution.

Aashish Chandorkar would like to thank his wife, Sudharani, and his family for the support they extended by not demanding his time. It enabled him to work long hours in researching and writing. Aashish would also like to thank his boss, Brajendra Navnit, India's Permanent Representative and Ambassador to the WTO, for his insights into the challenges of governance as well as for his understanding.

Suraj Sudhir would like to thank his wife, Eri, and his family for their support and encouragement through these difficult months of effort. He dedicates this effort to the memory of his father, A.P. Sudhir, whose lifetime of public service inspired his effort on digging into the data behind this topic.

Last but not the least, the authors express their gratitude to the readers of this book. Your faith is our booster dose of motivation.

NOTES

Hope Dawns

1. 'Laga Bhi Di…: What PM Modi Told Nurse after Receiving Covid-19 Vaccine at AIIMS', *India Today*, 1 March 2021, https://bit.ly/3VvnkGR. Accessed on 17 October 2022.
2. @PBNS_India, Twitter, 1 March 2021, 9.57 p.m., https://bit.ly/3E68Iam. Accessed on 17 October 2022.
3. @narendramodi, Twitter, 1 March 2021, 7.06 a.m., https://bit.ly/3yNbEWl. Accessed on 17 October 2022.

Chapter 1: Dark Clouds Engulf the World

1. Smil, Vaclav, *Global Catastrophes and Trends: The Next Fifty Years*, MIT Press, 2012, p. 46.
2. Gates, Bill, 'We're Not Ready for the Next Epidemic', Gates Notes, 18 March 2015, https://gatesnot.es/3CFvQua. Accessed on 17 October 2022.
3. Konyndyk, Jeremy, 'Donald Trump, Master of Disaster', *Politico Magazine*, 1 March 2017, https://politi.co/3S96bQe. Accessed on 17 October 2022.
4. Webster, Robert G., 'The Flu Expert Who Predicted a Pandemic: "Millions of People Would Die"', 14 July 2020, *Newsroom*, https://bit.ly/3yL9vdN. Accessed on 17 October 2022.
5. From an interview with Dr Krishna Ella, managing director, Bharat Biotech, conducted by Aashish Chandorkar on 28 July 2022.
6. 'Health Security: Combating Pandemics', Carnegie India YouTube, 31 January 2020, https://bit.ly/3TpU9TU. Accessed on 17 October 2022.
7. Ma, Josephine, 'Coronavirus: China's First Confirmed Covid-19 Case Traced Back to November 17', *South China Morning Post*, 13 March 2020, https://bit.ly/3rYqR2S. Accessed on 17 October 2022.
8. Stephanie, Hegarty, 'The Chinese Doctor Who Tried to Warn Others about Coronavirus', BBC, 6 February 2020, https://bbc.in/3TuDRsX. Accessed on 17 October 2022.
9. Zimmer, Carl, Benjamin Mueller and Chris Buckley, 'First Known Covid

Case Was Vendor at Wuhan Market, Scientist Says', *The New York Times*, 18 November 2021, https://nyti.ms/3U6tE6B. Accessed on 7 November 2022.

10. Ibid.
11. Ibid.
12. 'Archived: WHO Timeline-Covid-19', World Health Organization, 27 April 2020, https://bit.ly/3S87gbl. Accessed on 17 October 2022.
13. Ibid.
14. Cohen, Jon, 'Chinese Researchers Reveal Draft Genome of Virus Implicated in Wuhan Pneumonia Outbreak', *Science*, 11 January 2020, https://bit.ly/3WY0DMh. Accessed on 17 October 2022.
15. 'Archived: WHO Timeline-Covid-19', World Health Organization, 27 April 2020, https://bit.ly/3S87gbl. Accessed on 17 October 2022.
16. Chan, Jasper Fuk-Woo, et al., 'A Familial Cluster of Pneumonia Associated with the 2019 Novel Coronavirus Indicating Person-to-Person Transmission: A Study of a Family Cluster', *The Lancet*, vol. 395, no. 10223, 2020, pp. 514–23, https://bit.ly/3MzRlBj. Accessed on 17 October 2022.
17. @WHO, Twitter, 12 January 2020, 10.01 p.m., https://bit.ly/3CCsF6v. Accessed on 17 October 2022.
18. @WHO, Twitter, 14 January 2020, 4.48 p.m., https://bit.ly/3D0GjC2. Accessed on 17 October, 2022.
19. 'Naming the Coronavirus Disease (COVID-19) and the Virus That Causes It', World Health Organization, https://bit.ly/3ghwh6z. Accessed on 18 October 2022.
20. Handley, Erin, 'From Wuhan to Australia: A Timeline of Key Events in the Spread of the Deadly Coronavirus', ABC News, 6 April 2020, https://ab.co/3VN22Vx. Accessed on 18 October 2022.
21. Unnithan, P.S. Gopikrishnan, 'Kerala Reports First Confirmed Coronavirus Case in India', *India Today*, 31 January 2020, https://bit.ly/3MFxRLN. Accessed on 18 October 2022.
22. 'India's First Coronavirus Death Confirmed in Karnataka', *The Economic Times*, 13 March 2020, https://bit.ly/3CNr91M. Accessed on 18 October.
23. Gandhi-Mody, Priyam, *A Nation to Protect: Leading India Through the Crisis*, Rupa Publications, 2022, p. 23.
24. Ghosh, Abantika, Ananthakrishnan G. and Astha Saxena, 'COVID-19 Latest Updates March 23: 20 States, UTs Under Lockdown as Cases Mount to 433', *The Indian Express*, 23 March 2020, https://bit.ly/3gfej4F. Accessed on 18 October 2022.
25. 'PM Modi Calls for 'Janata Curfew' on March 22 from 7 AM-9 PM', *Business Line*, 20 March 2020, https://bit.ly/3TwHZIC. Accessed on 18 October 2022.

26. Gettleman, Jeffrey and Kai Schultz, 'Modi Orders 3-Week Total Lockdown for All 1.3 Billion Indians', *The New York Times*, by, 24 March 2020, https://nyti.ms/3rZeTWV. Accessed on 18 October 2022.
27. 'Text of PM's Address to the Nation on Vital Aspects Relating to the Menace of COVID-19', Press Information Bureau, Prime Minister's Office, 24 March 2022, https://bit.ly/3VxQGo7. Accessed on 18 October 2022.
28. 'Concerted Efforts of the Government, Industry and Multiple Stakeholders Turned the PPE Crisis into an Opportunity for India, Says Union Textiles Minister', Press Information Bureau, Ministry of Textiles, 11 December 2020, https://bit.ly/3CJ00gj. Accessed on 18 October 2022.
29. 'WHO Director-General's Opening Remarks at the Media Briefing on COVID-19-11 March 2020', World Health Organization, 11 March 2022, https://bit.ly/3EP8NzJ. Accessed on 18 October 2022.
30. 'Weekly Epidemiological Update on COVID-19 - 22 March 2022', World Health Organization, https://bit.ly/3zXYypH. Accessed on 8 November 2022.
31. 'India Situation', World Health Organization, https://bit.ly/3EaKyeS. Accessed on 8 November 2022.
32. 'CEPI to Fund Three Programmes to Develop Vaccines against the Novel Coronavirus, nCoV-2019', CEPI, 23 January 2020, https://bit.ly/3MGKC8w. Accessed on 18 October 2022.
33. Ravelo, Jenny Lei, and Sara Jerving, 'COVID-19 in 2020 — A Timeline of the Coronavirus Outbreak', Devex, https://bit.ly/3CI8sw5. Accessed on 18 October 2022.

Chapter 2: The One Millilitre Elixir

1. Kelly, Heath, 'The Classical Definition of a Pandemic Is Not Elusive', *Bulletin of the World Health Organization*, vol. 89, no. 7, 2011, pp. 540–1, https://bit.ly/3MEllvO. Accessed on 18 October 2022.
2. Watts, Edwards, and Zócalo Public Square, 'What Rome Learned from the Deadly Antonine Plague of 165 A.D.', *Smithsonian Magazine*, 28 April 2020, https://bit.ly/3ENwGYu. Accessed on 18 October 2022.
3. LePan, Nicholas, 'Visualizing the History of Pandemics', Visual Capitalist, 14 March 2020, https://bit.ly/3D6Y6rl. Accessed on 18 October 2022.
4. Ibid.
5. 'Study India's Earlier Pandemics — Collective Memory Holds Vital Lessons', *The Times of India*, 8 May 2021, https://bit.ly/3s4E0HM. Accessed on 18 October 2022.
6. Patel, Dhaval, 'Importance of Free Ration Supplies During Covid-19: Lessons From The 1918 Spanish Flu', *Swarajya Magazine*, 2 July 2021,

https://bit.ly/3CFHwxg. Accessed on 18 October 2022.

7. Baxby, Derrick, 'Edward Jenner's Inquiry; A Bicentenary Analysis', *Vaccine*, vol. 17, no. 4, 1999, pp. 301–7.
8. Fitzpatrick, Kieran, 'What Can Edward Jenner's Smallpox Vaccine Tell Us about Covid?', RTE, 13 January 2021, https://bit.ly/3NLZ6Vf. Accessed on 8 November 2022.
9. 'Edward Jenner, FRS FRCPE, The Father of Vaccination', The College of Physicians of Philadelphia, https://bit.ly/3UDdUIj. Accessed on 3 November 2022.
10. Klein, S., Irene Schöneberg and Gerard Krause, 'The Historical Development of Immunization in Germany. From Compulsory Smallpox Vaccination to a National Action Plan on Immunization', *Federal Health Bulletin - Health Research - Health Protection*, vol. 55, no. 11–12, 2012, pp. 1512–23.
11. 'United Kingdom Vaccination Act 1853', The Health Foundation - Policy Navigator, https://bit.ly/3s1HrPl. Accessed on 18 October 2022.
12. Wood, Margaret E., 'Biting Back', Science History Institute, 12 August 2016, https://bit.ly/2jpoGlF. Accessed on 18 October 2022.
13. Munthe, Axel, *The Story of San Michele*, John Murray, 1929.
14. Rowling, Megan, 'UN Aid Chief on Coronavirus: "No One Is Safe Until Everyone Is Safe"', World Economic Forum, 26 March 2020, https://bit.ly/3yNOHSI. Accessed on 18 October 2022.
15. 'How Are Vaccines Developed', World Health Organization, 8 December 2020, https://bit.ly/3MCILlp. Accessed on 18 October 2022.
16. Bloom, Barry R., and Paul-Henri Lambert (eds), *The Vaccine Book*, Academic Press, 2016, pp. 543–60.
17. 'History of the Measles Vaccine', World Health Organization, https://bit.ly/3UBliEb. Accessed on 14 November 2022.
18. Gillespie, Claire, 'How Many People Die from the Flu Each Year', *Health*, 25 October 2022, https://bit.ly/3CzdHhy. Accessed on 18 October 2022.
19. Prabhu, Maya, 'Mumps: The Story of the Second Fastest Vaccine Ever Developed', Gavi, 22 April 2022, https://bit.ly/3CIobLS. Accessed on 18 October 2022.
20. Michelson, Andrea, 'How the Coronavirus Vaccine Development Compares to Other Shots in History', *Business Insider*, 20 November 2020, https://bit.ly/3gdmePS. Accessed on 18 October 2022.
21. 'Commemorating Smallpox Eradication – A Legacy of Hope, for COVID-19 and Other Diseases', World Health Organization, 8 May 2020, https://bit.ly/3NMwECI. Accessed on 8 November 2022.
22. 'World Health Aides Mark Eradication of Smallpox', *The New York Times*, 9 May 1980, p. 7.

23. Ghosh, Pallabh, 'Rinderpest Virus Has Been Wiped Out, Scientists Say', BBC, 14 October 2010, https://bbc.in/3geRrSK. Accessed on 18 October 2022.
24. McNeil, Donald G., Jr., 'Rinderpest, Scourge of Cattle, Is Vanquished', *The New York Times*, 27 June 2011, https://nyti.ms/3Txah5N. Accessed on 18 October 2022.
25. 'Moderna Announces Funding Award from CEPI to Accelerate Development of Messenger RNA (mRNA) Vaccine against Novel Coronavirus', *Bloomberg*, 23 January 2020, https://bloom.bg/3ggmSw4. Accessed on 18 October 2022.
26. Dunn, Andrew, 'The First Trial of a Potential Coronavirus Vaccine Just Started in Washington State. It Will Take at Least a Year to Know If the Vaccine Works', *Business Insider*, 16 March 2020, https://bit.ly/3ggDgN9. Accessed on 18 October 2022.
27. 'Oxford Team to Begin Novel Coronavirus Vaccine Research', University of Oxford, 7 February 2020, https://bit.ly/3VABXsl. Accessed on 18 October.
28. Jacobs, Jennifer, and Drew Armstrong, 'Trump's "Operation Warp Speed" Aims to Rush Coronavirus Vaccine', *Bloomberg*, 29 April 2020, https://bloom.bg/3SaPyE2. Accessed on 18 October 2022.
29. Wise, Alana, 'Trump Promises "Warp Speed" Coronavirus Vaccine Effort with New Program', NPR, 15 May 2020, https://n.pr/3CHXHtI. Accessed on 18 October 2022.
30. Jacobs, Jennifer, and Drew Armstrong, 'Trump's "Operation Warp Speed" Aims to Rush Coronavirus Vaccine', *Bloomberg*, 29 April 2020, https://bloom.bg/3SaPyE2. Accessed on 18 October 2022.
31. Sanger, David E., 'Trump Seeks Push to Speed Vaccine, Despite Safety Concerns', *The New York Times*, 29 April 2020, https://nyti.ms/3CDZekx. Accessed on 18 October 2022.
32. From an interview with Dr Peter Hotez, dean for the National School of Tropical Medicine, Baylor College of Medicine Houston, US, conducted by Abhinav Joshi, Aashish Chandorkar and Suraj Sudhir on 5 April 2022.
33. Ibid.

Chapter 3: The Race to the Finish

1. 'Explaining Operation Warp Speed', U.S. Department of Health and Human Services, https://bit.ly/3Tf6drd. Accessed on 19 October 2022.
2. Wise, Alana, 'Trump Promises "Warp Speed" Coronavirus Vaccine Effort with New Programme', NPR, 15 May 2020, https://n.pr/3TA1S1s. Accessed on 19 October 2022.
3. Robbins, Rebecca, and Sheryl Gay Stolberg, 'Moderna Backs Down in Its Vaccine Patent Fight with the N.I.H.', *The New York Times*, 17 December

2021, https://nyti.ms/3CJQd9F. Accessed on 19 October 2022.

4. 'Johnson & Johnson Announces Collaboration with U.S. Department of Health & Human Services to Accelerate Development of a Potential Novel Coronavirus Vaccine', Johnson & Johnson, 11 February 2020, https://bit.ly/3VyyE5f. Accessed on 19 October 2022.
5. 'Sanofi Joins Forces with U.S. Department of Health and Human Services to Advance a Novel Coronavirus Vaccine', Sanofi, 18 February 2020, https://bit.ly/3S75G9D. Accessed on 19 October 2022.
6. Chalmers, John, and Kate Abnett, 'EU Rejects Accusations of "Vaccine Nationalism"', Reuters, 9 March 2021, https://reut.rs/3CMiDQk. Accessed on 19 October 2022.
7. 'Coronavirus: Commission Offers Financing to Innovative Vaccines Company CureVac', European Commission, 16 March 2020, https://bit.ly/3gd2v2J. Accessed on 19 October 2022.
8. Findlay, Stephanie, Michael Peel and Donato Paolo Mancini, 'India Blocks Vaccine Exports in Blow to Dozens of Nations', *Financial Times*, 25 March 2021, https://on.ft.com/3ML7nIQ. Accessed on 19 October 2022.
9. Florko, Nicholas, 'Trump Announces a Formal Freeze on WHO Funding, Pending an Investigation', STAT, 14 April 2020, https://bit.ly/3TAio1Q. Accessed on 19 October 2022.
10. 'World Leaders Pledge Billions for Coronavirus Vaccine', Deutsche Welle, 4 May 2020, https://bit.ly/3TxeAhH. Accessed on 19 October 2022.
11. From study of Advance Purchase Agreements of the European Commission.
12. From an interview with Dr Balram Bhargava, director of ICMR, conducted by Aashish Chandorkar on 24 April 2022.

Chapter 4: Vaccinations in India: A Modern History

1. 'Polio-Free Countries', Polio Global Eradication Initiative, https://bit.ly/3VCf9Zg. Accessed on 19 October 2022.
2. John, T. Jacob, and Vipin M. Vashishtha, 'Eradicating Poliomyelitis: India's Journey from Hyperendemic to Polio-Free Status', *The Indian Journal of Medical Research*, vol. 137, no. 5, 2013, pp. 881–94, https://bit.ly/3MJRFxn. Accessed on 19 October 2022.
3. Lahariya, Chandrakant, 'A Brief History of Vaccines and Vaccination in India', *The Indian Journal of Medical Research*, vol. 139, no. 4, 2014, pp. 491–511, https://bit.ly/2G48oJJ. Accessed on 19 October 2022.
4. Dahlburg, John-Thor, 'Making an About-Face, India Now Courts Foreign Investment', *Los Angeles Times*, 15 December 1993, https://lat.ms/3Tz5AbK. Accessed on 19 October 2022.

5. 'Eleventh World Health Assembly', *Official Records of the World Health Organization*, no. 87, Minneapolis, 28 May–13 June 1958, Geneva, 1958, p. 525.
6. Ibid.
7. 'Development of the Global Smallpox Eradication Programme, 1958–1966', Louisiana State University, p. 36, https://bit.ly/3UDqyqL. Accessed on 3 November 2022.
8. Fenner, Frank, et al., *Smallpox and Its Eradication*, World Health Organization, 1988, p. 400.
9. 'India Engages the Pandemic', University of Michigan Library, https://bit.ly/3yQUwyS. Accessed on 19 October 2022.
10. Fenner, Frank, et al., *Smallpox and Its Eradication*, World Health Organization, 1988, p. 5.
11. Ibid. 467.
12. Ibid. 465.
13. Ibid. 469.
14. 'Reward Poster', University of Michigan Library, https://bit.ly/3CMg40P. Accessed on 19 October 2022.
15. 'India Engages the Pandemic', University of Michigan Library, https://bit.ly/3yQUwyS. Accessed on 19 October 2022.
16. *Road Transport Yearbook 2017–18 & 2018–19*, Ministry of Road Transport and Highways, Transport Research Wing, Government of India, https://bit.ly/3s4h3o4. Accessed on 19 October 2022.
17. Tucker, Jonathan B., *Scourge: The Once and Future Threat of Smallpox*, Atlantic Monthly Press, 2001.
18. 'Immunization', National Health Mission, https://bit.ly/3gjVCMZ. Accessed on 19 October 2022.
19. Ch 2.8, Health, 'Tenth Five-Year Plan 2022–07, https://bit.ly/3DYewmj. Accessed on 3 November 2022.
20. John, T. Jacob, 'Understanding the Scientific Basis of Preventing Polio by Immunization. Pioneering Contributions from India', *Proceedings of the Indian National Science Academy*, 2003, pp. 393–422.
21. Ratnaswamy, L., T.J. John and M. Jadhav, 'Paralytic Poliomyelitis: Clinical and Virological Studies', *Indian Pediatrics*, vol. 10, no. 7, 1973, pp. 443–7.
22. Neelakantan, Vivek, 'Tuberculosis Control in Postcolonial South India and Southeast Asia: Fractured Sovereignties in International Health 1948–1960', *Wellcome Open Research*, 17 April 2018, https://bit.ly/3ScHwui. Accessed on 19 October 2022.
23. *National Strategic Plan for Tuberculosis: 2017–25 Elimination by 2025*, Ministry of Health and Family Welfare, 2017, https://bit.ly/3ggLfcX.

Accessed on 19 October 2022.

24. John, T.J., 'Problems with Oral Polio Vaccine in India', *Indian Pediatrics*, vol. 9, no. 5, 1972, pp. 252–6.
25. John, T.J., 'The Golden Jubilee of Vaccination against Poliomyelitis', *The Indian Journal of Medical Research*, vol. 119, no. 1, 2004, pp. 1–17.
26. Workman, Daniel, 'Drugs and Medicine Exports by Country', World's Top Exports, https://bit.ly/3CK18jH. Accessed on 19 October 2022.
27. 'PM Narendra Modi Launches Rotavirus Vaccine Developed in India', NDTV, 9 March 2015, https://bit.ly/3eIoKgK. Accessed on 19 October 2022.
28. From an interview with Dr Krishna Ella, managing director, Bharat Biotech, conducted by Aashish Chandorkar on 28 July 2022.
29. From an interview with senior Gavi officials, conducted by Aashish Chandorkar in June 2022.
30. 'Historic Partnership between Gavi and India to Save Millions of Lives', Gavi, 6 January 2016, https://bit.ly/3Vw7dZA. Accessed on 19 October 2022.
31. From an interview with senior Gavi officials, conducted by Aashish Chandorkar in June 2022.
32. From an interview with senior Gavi officials, conducted by Aashish Chandorkar in June 2022; 'Dr. Seth Berkley, CEO of Gavi, the Vaccine Alliance, Calls on PM', Narendra Modi, 6 January 2016, https://bit.ly/3TtH3VC. Accessed on 19 October 2022.

Chapter 5: Making Dhanvantari, Sushruta and Charaka Proud

1. Krishnan, Murali, 'Why the World Depends on India's Vaccine Production to Beat COVID', *DW*, 4 June 2021, https://bit.ly/3MIgMkh. Accessed on 20 October 2022.
2. Sarkale, Prasad, et al., 'First Isolation of SARS-CoV-2 from Clinical Samples in India', *The Indian Journal of Medical Research*, vol. 151, no. 2–3, 2020, pp. 244–50, https://bit.ly/3Dclp2P. Accessed on 20 October 2022.
3. Sapkal, Gajanan N., et al., 'Inactivated COVID-19 Vaccine BBV152/COVAXIN Effectively Neutralizes Recently Emerged B.1.1.7 Variant of SARS-CoV-2', *Journal of Travel Medicine*, vol. 28, no. 4, 2021, https://bit.ly/3yQcdhR. Accessed on 20 October 2022.
4. From an interview with Dr Krishna Ella, managing director, Bharat Biotech, conducted by Aashish Chandorkar on 28 July 2022.
5. Jha, Durgesh Nandan, 'Fewer Cases, But India Becomes 5th Country to Isolate Coronavirus', *The Times of India*, 14 March 2020, https://bit.

ly/3CF0J20. Accessed on 20 October 2022.

6. Ibid.
7. Pulla, Priyanka, 'Ray of Hope: Government Eases Restrictions on Indian COVID-19 Research', *The Wire*, 24 March 2020, https://bit.ly/3SeNk6v. Accessed on 20 October 2022.
8. 'India's S&T Institutions Raise their Game Against COVID-19', Press Information Bureau, Ministry of Science and Technology, 6 April 2020, https://bit.ly/3Thy5Ls. Accessed on 20 October 2022.
9. Arnimesh, Shanker, '20 Indian Institutes Working to Find Covid-19 Vaccine, IITs Focused on Portable Ventilators', *The Print*, 27 March 2020, https://bit.ly/3gotpF1. Accessed on 20 October 2022.
10. Ibid.
11. From interviews with senior Gavi officials conducted by Aashish Chandorkar in June 2022.
12. 'PM Narendra Modi Uses Homemade Face Mask during CMs Meeting on Covid-19', *The Times of India*, 11 April 2020, https://bit.ly/3gbJGNk. Accessed on 20 October 2022.
13. Gandhi-Mody, Priyam, *A Nation to Protect: Leading India through the Covid Crisis*, Rupa Publications, 2022, p. 80.
14. Jesline, Joshy, et al., 'The Plight of Migrants during COVID-19 and the Impact of Circular Migration in India: A Systematic Review', *Humanities and Social Sciences Communications*, vol. 8, no. 231, 2021, https://go.nature.com/3EXafAj. Accessed on 20 October 2022.
15. From interviews with Ministry of Health and Family Welfare officials conducted by Aashish Chandorkar on 28 April 2022.
16. 'India's S&T Institutions Raise their Game Against COVID-19', Press Information Bureau, Ministry of Science and Technology, 6 April 2020, https://bit.ly/3Thy5Ls. Accessed on 20 October 2022.
17. Ibid.
18. Ibid.
19. Ibid.
20. Kames, Jacob, et al., 'Sequence Analysis of SARS-CoV-2 Genome Reveals Features Important for Vaccine Design', *Scientific Reports*, vol. 10, no. 1, 2020, https://bit.ly/3TxK3Ag. Accessed on 20 October 2022.
21. 'DNA Sequencing Fact Sheet', National Human Genome Research Institute, https://bit.ly/2IyQdOA. Accessed on 20 October 2022.
22. 'Gujarat Institute Identifies 3 New Mutations of Novel Coronavirus', *India Today*, 17 April 2020, https://bit.ly/3eLXEp0. Accessed on 20 October 2022.
23. 'About CSIR', Council of Scientific and Industrial Research, https://bit.ly/3DeErpr. Accessed on 20 October 2022.

24. 'CSIR Submits 53 Genome Sequences of Coronavirus to Global Body; to Share 450 More by May 15', *The Economic Times*, 7 May 2020, https://bit.ly/3SeZigA. Accessed on 20 October 2022.
25. Scimago Institutions Rankings, https://bit.ly/3Sg6lFC. Accessed on 20 October 2022.
26. 'About CSIR', Council of Scientific and Industrial Research, https://bit.ly/3DeErpr. Accessed on 20 October 2022.
27. 'Inactivated Virus Vaccine in Focus for Novel Coronavirus', Press Information Bureau, Ministry of Science and Technology, 16 April 2020, https://bit.ly/3MMRTUz. Accessed on 20 October 2022.
28. 'PM Chairs a Meeting of the Task Force on Corona Vaccine Development, Drug Discovery, Diagnosis and Testing', Press Information Bureau, Prime Minister's Office, 5 May 2020, https://bit.ly/3yUsGSm. Accessed on 20 October 2022.
29. From an interview with unnamed Prime Minister's Office officials conducted by Aashish Chandorkar on 20 March 2022.
30. Mazzucato, Mariana, *The Entrepreneurial State*, Penguin Books, 2013. The book argues that the private sector only finds the courage to invest after an entrepreneurial state has made the high-risk investments.
31. 'Indian Council of Medical Research (ICMR) Partners with Bharat Biotech International Limited (BBIL) for Developing Indigenous COVID-19 Vaccine', Indian Council of Medical Research, 9 May 2022, https://bit.ly/3saEIDp. Accessed on 20 October 2022.
32. 'Funding and Manufacturing Boost for UK Vaccine Programme', Department for Business, Energy and Industrial Strategy, Government of UK, 17 May 2020, https://bit.ly/3goNYBi. Accessed on 20 October 2022.
33. 'Coronavirus: EU Supports Vaccine Research with Additional €100 Million', European Commission, 22 July 2020, https://bit.ly/3TSZHqj. Accessed on 20 October 2022.
34. '$17M Shot in the Arm for UQ's COVID-19 Vaccine Research', The University of Queensland, Australia, 22 March 2020, https://bit.ly/3SeQo2v. Accessed on 20 October 2022.
35. 'About Us | Introduction', Serum Institute of India, https://bit.ly/2QHNmbz. Accessed on 20 October 2022.
36. 'AstraZeneca and the University of Oxford Announce Landmark Agreement for COVID-19 Vaccine', AstraZeneca, 30 April 2020, https://bit.ly/3CPUsAH. Accessed on 20 October 2022.
37. Roy, Abhirup, and Euan Rocha, 'How One Indian Company Could Be World's Door to a COVID-19 Vaccine', Reuters, 22 May 2020, https://reut.rs/3eLw7ny. Accessed on 20 October 2022.

38. 'AstraZeneca Takes Next Steps towards Broad and Equitable Access to the University of Oxford's COVID-19 Vaccine', AstraZeneca, 4 June 2020, https://bit.ly/3VEMKSz. Accessed on 20 October 2022.
39. Marandi, Rosemary, and Raj Kumar Sharma, 'Coronavirus Tests India's Vaccine Makers in R&D Capability', Nikkei Asia, 21 May 2020, https://s.nikkei.com/3gkqGfJ. Accessed on 20 October 2022.
40. From an interview with Ministry of Health and Family Welfare officials conducted by Aashish Chandorkar on 28 April 2022.
41. From an interview with Sanjeev Navangul, managing director and CEO, Bharat Serums and Vaccines Ltd, conducted by Aashish Chandorkar and Suraj Sudhir on 22 March 2022.
42. 'Health Security: Combating Pandemics, Carnegie India Global Technology Summit 2019', YouTube, 31 January 2020, https://bit.ly/3TpU9TU. Accessed on 17 October 2022.
43. From an interview with Ministry of Health and Family Welfare officials conducted by Aashish Chandorkar on 28 April 2022.
44. Bhargava, Balram, 'We Need an Enabling Ecosystem for Development of Vaccines, Studies on New Diseases', *The Indian Express*, 4 June 2020, https://bit.ly/3FFVgel. Accessed on 3 November 2022.
45. From interview with PMO officials conducted by Aashish Chandorkar on 20 March 2022.
46. 'To Ramp Up Vaccine Output, Government Pumps in Funds', *The Times of India*, 17 April 2021, https://bit.ly/3Tfr8u9. Accessed on 20 October 2022.
47. 'PM's Address to the Nation on 12.5.2020', PM India, 12 May 2020, https://bit.ly/3yThuVW. Accessed on 20 October 2022.
48. 'India's 1st COVID-19 Vaccine – COVAXIN™, Developed by Bharat Biotech Gets DCGI Approval for Phase I & II Human Clinical Trials', Bharat Biotech, 15 July 2020, https://bit.ly/3DlHLzb. Accessed on 20 October 2022.
49. 'India Races to Release First Indigenous COVID-19 Vaccine by August 15', *Hindustan Times*, 3 July 2020, https://bit.ly/3goezy8. Accessed on 20 October 2022.
50. Kumar, Sanjay, 'Scientists Scoff at Indian Agency's Plan to Have COVID-19 Vaccine Ready for Use Next Month', *Science*, 6 July 2020, https://bit.ly/3yWGSKu. Accessed on 20 October 2022.
51. Sharma, Neetu Chandra, 'Haven't Set 15 Aug as Deadline for Covid-19 Vaccine, Says ICMR', *Mint*, 6 July 2020, https://bit.ly/3TiPtj0. Accessed on 20 October 2022.
52. 'English Rendering of PM's Address at the Launch of High Throughput COVID-19 Testing Facilities at 3 ICMR Labs', Press Information Bureau, Prime Minister's Office, 27 July 2000, https://bit.ly/3CHEOqW. Accessed

on 20 October 2022.

53. 'Aatmanirbhar Bharat Has Become a 'Mantra' for the 130 Crore Indians Today: PM Modi during 74th Independence Day', Narendra Modi, 15 August 2020, https://bit.ly/3yVi99H. Accessed on 20 October 2022.
54. 'DBT's Response to COVID-19 | S&T Interventions for COVID-19', May 2021, https://bit.ly/3s7VqDm. Accessed on 20 October 2022.
55. Black, Steven, 'The Costs and Effectiveness of Large Phase III Pre-Licensure Vaccine Clinical Trials', *Expert Review of Vaccines*, vol. 14, no. 12, 2015, pp. 1543–8.
56. 'Human Trials for COVID-19 Vaccine Initiated in India with 1,000 Volunteers: ICMR', *The Economic Times*, 14 July 2020, https://bit.ly/3yXfR9T. Accessed on 20 October 2022.
57. 'Serum Institute of India Seeks DCGI Permission for Phase 2/3 Clinical Trials of Oxford's COVID "Vaccine"', *The Economic Times*, 25 July 2020, https://bit.ly/3SeVvjd. Accessed on 20 October 2022.
58. From an interview with Sanjeev Navangul, managing director and CEO, Bharat Serums and Vaccines Ltd, conducted by Aashish Chandorkar and Suraj Sudhir on 22 March 2022.
59. 'COVID-19 Update: Serum Institute of India to Start Phase 2 and 3 Human Clinical Trials of Oxford Vaccine Candidate', *The Economic Times*, 3 August 2020, https://bit.ly/3gfTqpP. Accessed on 20 October 2022.
60. Ray, Meenakshi, 'Price, Trial Timeline of Serum Institute's Covid-19 Vaccine', *Hindustan Times*, 22 July 2020, https://bit.ly/3s8ty1M. Accessed on 20 October 2022.
61. 'Serum Institute of India Seeks DCGI Permission for Phase 2/3 Clinical Trials of Oxford's COVID "Vaccine"', *The Economic Times*, 25 July 2020, https://bit.ly/3SeVvjd. Accessed on 20 October 2022.
62. Ibid.
63. 'Panel Recommends Serum Institute's Name for Phase 2, 3 Human Clinical Trials of Oxford Vaccine Candidate', *The Economic Times*, 31 July 2020, https://bit.ly/3eHj1rB. Accessed on 20 October 2022.
64. Chandna, Himani, 'SII Proposes 1,600 Subjects in 20 Indian Cities for Oxford Vaccine Trials, Govt to Decide Today', *The Print*, 31 July 2020, https://bit.ly/3UjXd4b. Accessed on 3 November 2022.
65. Ibid.
66. Thacker, Teena, 'Serum Institute of India Gets Approval to Start Human Trials for Oxford Vaccine', *The Economic Times*, 1 August 2020, https://bit.ly/3gnAqFU. Accessed on 20 October 2022.
67. From an interview with Ministry of Health and Family Welfare officials, conducted by Aashish Chandorkar on 28 April 2022.

68. Gettleman, Jeffrey, 'Indian Billionaires Bet Big on Head Start in Coronavirus Vaccine Race', *The New York Times*, 1 August 2020, https://nyti.ms/3gbT2Zs. Accessed on 20 October 2022.
69. Nathan-Kazis, Josh, 'Novavax Announces Deals to Sell Covid-19 Vaccine in India, Japan, and Low-Income Countries', Barron's, 7 August 2020, https://bit.ly/3SbTjsF. Accessed on 20 October 2022.
70. 'Up to 100 Million COVID-19 Vaccine Doses to Be Made Available for Low- and Middle-Income Countries As Early As 2021', Gavi, 7 August 2020, https://bit.ly/3sa32oV. Accessed on 20 October 2022.
71. 'Coronavirus Vaccine Update: Russia May Partner India for Producing Vaccines', *Business Standard*, 21 August 2020, https://bit.ly/3VKtN0T. Accessed on 20 October 2022.
72. From interview with Ministry of Health and Family Welfare officials conducted by Aashish Chandorkar on 28 April 2022.
73. Chatterji, Saubhadra, 'Covid-19 Vaccine Diplomacy in India's Outreach Plan', 31 August 2020, *Hindustan Times*, https://bit.ly/3CN51o3. Accessed on 20 October 2022.
74. 'Modi Offers India's COVID-19 Vaccine Capacity to "All Humanity"', Al Jazeera, 27 September 2020, Al Jazeera, https://bit.ly/3eIyB6i. Accessed on 20 October 2022.
75. Ravi, Vibha, 'India's Draft Guidelines for COVID-19 Vaccines Follow WHO, US Lead', Pink Sheet, 24 September 2020, https://bit.ly/3Shfg9K. Accessed on 20 October 2022.
76. 'Vaccines Candidates in Clinical Trials', Covid19 Vaccine Tracker, https://bit.ly/3yUdLHM. Accessed on 20 October 2022.
77. Chan-hyuk, Kim, 'Genexine to Give Up COVID-19 Vaccine Development', *Korea Biomedical Review*, 14 March 2022, https://bit.ly/3F8Q56n. Accessed on 24 October 2022.

Chapter 6: Beginning of the End?

1. 'Biopharma Leaders Unite to Stand with Science', Pfizer, 8 September 2020,, https://bit.ly/3MZFVXI. Accessed on 24 October 2022.
2. 'COVID-19 Vaccine Maker Pledge', Pfizer, https://bit.ly/3SrNNlP. Accessed on 24 October 2022.
3. Ibid.
4. 'Pfizer and BioNTech Announce Vaccine Candidate against COVID-19 Achieved Success in First Interim Analysis from Phase 3 Study', Pfizer, 9 November 2020, https://bit.ly/3VY95un. Accessed on 24 October 2022.
5. 'Early Data Show Moderna's Coronavirus Vaccine Is 94.5% Effective by Denise Grady', *The New York Times*, 16 November 2020, https://nyti.

ms/3TTVnGW. Accessed on 24 October 2022.

6. Robbins, Rebecca, and Benjamin Mueller, 'AstraZeneca's Coronavirus Vaccine, Easy and Cheap to Produce, Appears Effective', *The New York Times*, 23 November 2020, https://nyti.ms/3snq383. Accessed on 24 October 2022.
7. Ibid.
8. Dey, Sushmi, 'Serum Institute Readies 40m Doses of Covid Vaccine under "At Risk" Manufacturing, Stockpiling Licence', *The Times of India*, 13 November 2020, https://bit.ly/3Famyt0. Accessed on 24 October 2022.
9. Karmali, Naazneen, 'Serum Institute of India Takes a Multipronged Approach in Quest to Produce World's First Covid-19 Vaccines', *Forbes*, 7 October 2020, https://bit.ly/3D8OkUf. Accessed on 25 October 2022.
10. 'Bharat Biotech Starts Phase III Trials for COVAXIN', Bharat Biotech, 16 November 2020, https://bit.ly/3FiW0Gb. Accessed on 25 October 2022.
11. Das, Sohini, 'Bharat Biotech Starts Covaxin's At-Risk Manufacturing; Expanding Capacity', *Business Standard*, 24 October 2020, https://bit.ly/3FhQUd6. Accessed on 25 October 2022.
12. 'FDA Takes Key Action in Fight against COVID-19 by Issuing Emergency Use Authorization for First COVID-19 Vaccine', U.S. Food and Drug Administration, 11 December 2020, https://bit.ly/3D7ZUio. Accessed on 25 October 2022.
13. Ibid.
14. 'FDA Takes Additional Action in Fight against COVID-19 by Issuing Emergency Use Authorization for Second COVID-19 Vaccine', U.S. Food and Drug Administration, 18 December 2020, https://bit.ly/3stmVaL. Accessed on 25 October 2022.
15. Ibid.
16. 'AstraZeneca's COVID-19 Vaccine Authorised for Emergency Supply in the UK', AstraZeneca, 30 December 2020, https://bit.ly/3SAZ2ss. Accessed on 25 October 2022.
17. Ibid.
18. 'The Subject Expert Committee (SEC) of Central Drugs Standards Control Organisation (CDSCO) Makes Recommendations in Respect of Accelerated Approval Process Request of M/s Serum Institute of India and M/s Bharat Biotech International Ltd As Well As About Phase III Trials of M/s Cadila Healthcare Ltd', Press Information Bureau, Ministry of Health and Family Welfare, 2 January 2021, https://bit.ly/3fdmf69. Accessed on 25 October 2022.
19. 'Press Statement by the Drugs Controller General of India (DCGI) on Restricted Emergency Approval of COVID-19 Virus Vaccine', Press

Information Bureau, Ministry of Health and Family Welfare, 3 January 2021, https://bit.ly/3DypTkx. Accessed on 25 October 2022.

20. 'Coronavirus: India Approves Vaccines from Bharat Biotech and Oxford/ AstraZeneca', BBC, 3 January2021, https://bbc.in/3TXCpzn. Accessed on 25 October 2022.
21. Banerjea, Aparna, 'Covid Vaccine: Covaxin Phase-3 Efficacy Data by March, Says Bharat Biotech CMD, *Mint*, 4 January 2021, https://bit.ly/3zES3rU. Accessed on 3 November 2022.
22. 'AZD1222 Oxford Phase III Trials Interim Analysis Results Published in the Lancet', AstraZeneca, 8 December 2020. Accessed on 25 October 2022.
23. 'Pfizer and BioNTech Conclude Phase 3 Study of COVID-19 Vaccine Candidate, Meeting All Primary Efficacy Endpoints', Pfizer, 18 November 2020, https://bit.ly/3gKHjl6. Accessed on 25 October 2022.
24. 'About Our Landmark Trial', Pfizer, https://bit.ly/3Dz5hbQ. Accessed on 25 October 2022.
25. Masih, Niha, 'India Approves Two Vaccines As It Prepares for Massive Immunization Push', *The Washington Post*, 3 January 2020, https://wapo.st/3SwhZwk. Accessed on 25 October 2022.
26. Pulla, Priyanka, 'Scientists Criticize 'Rushed' Approval of Indian COVID-19 Vaccine without Efficacy Data', *Science*, 6 January 2021, https://bit.ly/3SDlEZp. Accessed on 25 October 2022.
27. Ibid.
28. Pai, Nitin, 'DCGI's Covaxin 'Approval' Is Political Jumla. It Reinforces Idea of Modi's Atmanirbhar Bharat', *The Print*, 5 January 2021, https://bit.ly/3U1odFH. Accessed on 25 October 2022.
29. From an interview with Dr Krishna Ella, managing director, Bharat Biotech, conducted by Aashish Chandorkar on 28 July 2022.
30. Oke, Yogini, and Shreya Shrivastava, 'How India's Regulatory Pitfalls Helped Covishield and Covaxin Get Rapid Approval', *The Print*, 8 January 2021, https://bit.ly/3DgjnOa. Accessed on 25 October 2022.
31. *The Gazette of India: PART II—Section 3—Sub-section (i)*, Ministry of Health and Family Welfare, 2019, p. 186, https://bit.ly/3TDo4bH. Accessed on 25 October 2022.
32. Ibid
33. Ibid.
34. Ibid.
35. Ibid.
36. Ibid.
37. Ibid., 185.
38. Oke, Yogini, and Shreya Shrivastava, 'How India's Regulatory Pitfalls Helped

Covishield and Covaxin Get Rapid Approval', *The Print*, 8 January 2021, https://bit.ly/3DgjnOa. Accessed on 25 October 2022.

39. *The Gazette of India: PART II—Section 3—Sub-section (i)*, Ministry of Health and Family Welfare, 2019, p. 186, https://bit.ly/3TDo4bH. Accessed on 25 October 2022.

Chapter 7: A Strategic Numbers Game

1. 'Covid-19 Weekly Epidemiological Update', World Health Organization, 20 December 2020, https://bit.ly/3Dylmyv. Accessed on 25 October 2022.
2. Ahluwalia, Shaina, and Roshan Abraham, 'Global COVID-19 Cases Surpass 100 Million As Nations Tackle Vaccine Shortages', Reuters, 27 January 2021, https://reut.rs/3gDgz5T. Accessed on 25 October 2022.
3. 'Herd Immunity and COVID-19: What You Need to Know', Mayo Clinic, https://mayocl.in/3ssUrxQ. Accessed on 25 October 2022.
4. Bolotin, Shelly, Sarah Wilson and Michelle Murti, 'Achieving and Sustaining Herd Immunity to SARS-CoV-2', *Canadian Medical Association Journal*, vol. 193, no. 28, 2021, p. E1089.
5. Winer, Stuart, 'Israel Will Reportedly Pay Much More than US, EU for Pfizer Coronavirus Vaccine', *Times of Israel*,16 November 2020, https://bit.ly/3zfMeAK. Accessed on 25 October 2022.
6. 'Pfizer CEO Hails "Obsessive" Netanyahu for Calling 30 Times to Seal Vaccine Deal', *Times of Israel*, 11 March 2021, https://bit.ly/3N7fOy4. Accessed on 25 October 2022.
7. Estrin, Daniel, 'Vaccines for Data: Israel's Pfizer Deal Drives Quick Rollout — And Privacy Worries', NPR, 31 January 2021, https://n.pr/3W47Gm3. Accessed on 25 October 2022.
8. Stevis-Gridneff, Matina, 'How Europe Sealed a Pfizer Vaccine Deal With Texts and Calls', *The New York Times*, 15 September 2021, https://nyti.ms/3TYEpau. Accessed on 25 October 2022.
9. Kresge, Naomi, and Riley Griffin, 'Pfizer to Cut Vaccine Shipments as Belgian Factory Renovated', *Bloomberg*, 16 January 2021, https://bloom.bg/3zdVmpK. Accessed on 25 October 2022.
10. Guarascio, Francesco, 'AstraZeneca to Miss Second-Quarter EU Vaccine Supply Target by Half - EU official', Reuters, 23 February 2021, https://reut.rs/3f823mk. Accessed on 25 October 2022.
11. @vonderleyen, Twitter, 14 April 2021, 5.39 p.m., https://bit.ly/3SDNk0a. Accessed on 25 October 2022.
12. 'Biden Administration Purchases Additional Doses of COVID-19 Vaccines from Pfizer and Moderna', HHS.gov, 11 February 2021, https://bit.

ly/3NbdTIP. Accessed on 25 October 2022.

13. Lupkin, Sydney, 'Defense Production Act Speeds up Vaccine Production', NPR, 13 March 2021, https://n.pr/3Dycs3Z. Accessed on 25 October 2022.
14. 'Six-Week Sprint Got Indian-Made AstraZeneca Vaccine Approved in Canada', USA News, 1 March 2021, https://bit.ly/3f9GCkL. Accessed on 25 October 2022.
15. Arora, Neha, and Rupam Jain, 'India Hopes U.S. Will Soon Ease Ban on Vaccine Material Exports', Reuters, 19 April 2021, https://reut.rs/3TUkTvZ. Accessed on 25 October 2022.
16. Normile, Dennis, 'Only 1% of Japan Is Fully Vaccinated against COVID-19. Is It Ready for the Olympics?', *Science*, 13 May 2021, https://bit.ly/3f1bggk. Accessed on 25 October 2022.
17. 'Pfizer and BioNTech to Supply Japan with 120 Million Doses of Their BNT162 mRNA-Based Vaccine Candidate', Pfizer, 31 July 2020, https://bit.ly/3SBorSS. Accessed on 25 October 2022.
18. Yamaguchi, Mari, 'In Venue Fit for Head of State, Japan PM Seeks Pfizer Doses', USA News, 23 July 2021, https://bit.ly/3zifc37. Accessed on 25 October 2022.
19. 'COVAX: CEPI's response to COVID-19', CEPI, https://bit.ly/3ssX2I6. Accessed on 25 October 2022.
20. From an interview with senior Gavi officials conducted by Aashish Chandorkar in June 2022.
21. Ibid.
22. Ibid.
23. Deutsch, Jillian, and Sarah Wheaton, 'How Europe Fell behind on Vaccines', *Politico*, 27 January 2021, https://politi.co/3TSf4z0. Accessed on 25 October 2022.
24. Dhamija, Anshul, 'The Ellas of Bharat Biotech: The Gift of the Jab', *Fortune India*, 7 May 2021, https://bit.ly/3swSbWs. Accessed on 25 October 2022.
25. Srivastava, Vanita, 'Zydus Cadila's Sharvil Patel: We Will Manufacture One Crore Doses per Month Initially', *MoneyControl*, 10 July 2021, https://bit.ly/3TZSg0a. Accessed on 25 October 2022.
26. 'Mission Covid Suraksha', Department of Biotechnology, Government of India, https://bit.ly/3SHYgcV. Accessed on 25 October 2022.
27. Ibid.
28. Ibid.
29. Bhalla, Vineet, 'Centre's Affidavits in SC Exposes Its Hollow Claims of Both Covid Vaccine Availability and Spending on Its Research and Development', *The Leaflet*, 18 July 2021, https://bit.ly/3D6BQfT. Accessed on 25 October 2022.

30. 'Coronavirus Covid-19 Vaccinations', Our World in Data, https://bit.ly/3TDFhlg. Accessed on 25 October 2022.
31. 'Role of CSIR', CSIR India, https://bit.ly/3N6tgSO. Accessed on 25 October 2022.
32. Collated from Government of India press releases.
33. Ibid.
34. Sheriff M., Kaunain, 'In a First, Centre Will Pay Rs 1,500 Crore to Reserve 30 Crore Doses of New Vaccine', *The Indian Express*, 4 June 2021, https://bit.ly/3TUqqCL. Accessed on 25 October 2022.
35. 'Centre Places Purchase Order for 5 Crore doses of COVID-19 Vaccine Corbevax', *The Hindu*, 5 February 2022, https://bit.ly/3fb0HXN. Accessed on 25 October 2022.
36. J.C., Anand, 'Zydus Cadila to Supply 1 Crore Doses of ZyCoV-D to Govt at Rs 265/Dose', *The Economic Times*, 8 November 2021, https://bit.ly/3zgjxUn. Accessed on 25 October 2022.
37. 'Update on COVID-19 Vaccine Availability in States/UTs', Press Information Bureau, Ministry of Health and Family Welfare, 30 September 2022, https://bit.ly/3fxcxMh. Accessed on 4 November 2022.
38. 'Serum Institute Produces over 100 Million Covishield Doses in June', *Business Standard*, 27 June 2021, https://bit.ly/3DyreYF. Accessed on 25 October 2022.
39. Leo, Leroy, 'Govt Aids Bharat Biotech with ₹65 Crore Grant, 3 PSUs' Support to Make Covaxin', *Mint*, 16 April 2021, https://bit.ly/3zgEezw. Accessed on 25 October 2022.
40. 'DBT-BIRAC supported ZyCoV-D developed by Zydus Cadila Receives Emergency Use Authorization', Press Information Bureau, Ministry of Science and Technology, 20 August 2021, https://bit.ly/3stv92u. Accessed on 25 October 2022.
41. Kirk, Ashley, Finbarr Sheehy and Cath Levett, 'Canada and UK among Countries with Most Vaccine Doses Ordered per Person', *The Guardian*, 29 January 2021, https://bit.ly/3N9IE0E. Accessed on 25 October 2022.
42. 'Coronavirus (COVID-19) Vaccinations', Our World in Data, https://bit.ly/3N98PVt. Accessed on 25 October 2022.
43. Co-WIN, Ministry of Health and Family Welfare, https://bit.ly/3TXOuVH. Accessed on 4 November 2022.
44. 'Covishield Vaccine Production Surpasses 1 Billion', Precision Vaccinations, 30 November 2021, https://bit.ly/3sOW9db. Accessed on 25 October 2022.
45. 'Pushing Boundaries to Deliver COVID-19 Vaccine across the Globe', AstraZeneca, https://bit.ly/3TFjzNE. Accessed on 25 October 2022.
46. Bown, Chad P., 'The US Was Quick to Produce COVID-19 Vaccines. Then

It Fell Behind', Peterson Institute for International Economics, 21 June 2022, https://bit.ly/3DvLWbs. Accessed on 25 October 2022.

47. 'White House Officials Say U.S. Has Exhausted Funds to Buy Potential Fourth Vaccine Dose for All Americans', *The Washington Post*, 22 March 2022, https://wapo.st/3W4sb1R. Accessed on 25 October 2022.

Chapter 8: Getting the Plumbing Right

1. K. Sambasiva, Sastri, *The Tantropakhyana*, Superintendent, Government Press, Trivandrum, 1938, p. 26.
2. Ehrlich, Paul R., *The Population Bomb*, Ballantine Books, 1968, p. 1.
3. Kritz, Fran, 'The Vaccine Passport Debate Actually Began In 1897 Over a Plague Vaccine', NPR, 8 April 2021, https://n.pr/3VZuiUZ. Accessed on 25 October 2022.
4. Paliwal, Ankur, 'Indian Swine Flu Vaccines Hit Market', DownToEarth, 14 July 2010, https://bit.ly/3DzAb3N. Accessed on 25 October 2022.
5. From interview with Dr Raman Gangakhedkar, retired head scientist of epidemiology and communicable diseases at the Indian Council of Medical Research, conducted by Aashish Chandorkar on 2 April 2022.
6. 'Estimates of Gross Domestic Product for the First Quarter (April-June) of 2020–21', Press Information Bureau, Ministry of Statistics and Programme Implementation, 31 August 2020, https://bit.ly/3DyCOTp. Accessed on 25 October 2022.
7. 'The States Subject List', Vakilbabu, https://bit.ly/3syJ4V4. Accessed on 25 October 2022.
8. From an interview with Sanjeev Navangul, managing director and CEO, Bharat Serums and Vaccines Ltd, conducted by Aashish Chandorkar and Suraj Sudhir on 22 March 2022.
9. Gandhi-Mody, Priyam, *A Nation to Protect: Leading India through the Covid Crisis*, Rupa Publications, 2022, p. 136.
10. Ibid.
11. Ibid. 137.
12. 'National Expert Group on Vaccine Administration for COVID-19 Deliberates on Strategy to Ensure COVID-19 Vaccines' Availability and its Delivery Mechanism', Press Information Bureau, Ministry of Health and Family Welfare, 12 August 2020, https://bit.ly/3FjrkEQ. Accessed on 25 October 2022.
13. 'WHO SAGE Roadmap for Prioritizing Uses of Covid-19 Vaccines in the Context of Limited Supply', World Health Organization, 13 November 2020, https://bit.ly/3VYiTol. Accessed on 25 October 2022.

14. Das, Sohini, and T.E. Narasimhan, 'Govt Begins Micro-Planning for Administering Covid-19 Vaccine to the Masses', *Business Standard*, 9 October 2020, https://bit.ly/3FiYEM1. Accessed on 25 October 2022.
15. Ibid.
16. Ibid.
17. '110 Million Children Vaccinated in the Country's First Polio Drive of the Decade', World Health Organization, 4 February 2021, https://bit.ly/3svIHKL. Accessed on 25 October 2022.
18. Das, Sohini, and T.E. Narasimhan, 'Govt Begins Micro-Planning for Administering Covid-19 Vaccine to the Masses', *Business Standard*, 9 October 2020, https://bit.ly/3FiYEM1. Accessed on 25 October 2022.
19. 'Status of IMR and MMR in India', Press Information Bureau, Ministry of Health and Family Welfare, 8 February 2022, https://bit.ly/3FjA1id. Accessed on 25 October 2022.
20. 'Universal Immunization Programme', Ministry of Health and Family Welfare, https://bit.ly/3DzAiMG. Accessed on 25 October 2022.
21. 'Ramping Up Cold Storage Facilities Critical As India Preps for COVID-19 Vaccine: Experts', *The Economic Times*, 8 October 2020, https://bit.ly/3UfECq6. Accessed on 4 November 2022.
22. 'Centre to Map Out Cold Chain Storage Facilities in Preparation for COVID-19 Vaccine Delivery', *The Economic Times*, 8 October 2020, https://bit.ly/3FAIder. Accessed on 25 October 2022.
23. 'Chhattisgarh Government Starts Preparation for COVID-19 Vaccination Drive', *The Economic Times*, 6 November 2020, https://bit.ly/3FjtVOQ. Accessed on 25 October 2022.
24. 'Constitution of State Steering Committee, State Task Force and District Task Force for COVID-19 Vaccination, 2020', Administration of Union Territory of Ladakh, Health and Medical Education Department, 30 November 2020, https://bit.ly/3TVJL6u. Accessed on 25 October 2022.
25. 'Goa Kick-Starts Preparation for Covid-19 Vaccine Roll-Out', *Business Insider India*, 2 December 2020, https://bit.ly/3W5DCGU. Accessed on 25 October 2022.
26. Madur, 'COVID 19 Vaccine Preparations in Karnataka', Karnataka.com, 25 November 2020, https://bit.ly/3W8TvfM. Accessed on 25 October 2022.
27. Sharma, Niharika, 'How Mumbai Airport Is Preparing to Transport the Covid-19 Vaccine', Quartz, 3 December 2020, https://bit.ly/3SGxNg1. Accessed on 25 October 2022.
28. 'Odisha Gets to Work on Covid-19 Vaccination', *The New Indian Express*, 24 October 2020, https://bit.ly/3FjBrcP. Accessed on 25 October 2022.
29. 'Coronavirus | Tamil Nadu Health Department Deputy Directors Told to

Prepare Micro Plan for COVID-19 Vaccination', *The Hindu*, 23 September 2020, https://bit.ly/3W2m2n5. Accessed on 25 October 2022.

30. 'PM Shri Narendra Modi Today Reviewed Preparedness of Covid-19 Vaccine Delivery, Distribution and Administration', Press Information Bureau, Prime Minister's Office, 20 November 2020, https://bit.ly/3TUqh2J. Accessed on 25 October 2022.
31. 'PM Chairs High Level Meeting with CMs to Review Status and Preparedness of COVID-19 Response and Management', Press Information Bureau, Prime Minister's Office, 24 November 2020, https://bit.ly/3D7DzSd. Accessed on 25 October 2022.
32. 'A New Digital Platform 'CO-WIN' Is Being Used for COVID-19 Vaccination Delivery', Press Information Bureau, Ministry of Health and Family Welfare, 8 December 2020, https://bit.ly/3DyRIsP. Accessed on 25 October 2022.
33. From interviews with unnamed officials from the Prime Minister's Office, conducted by Aashish Chandorkar on 20 March 2022.
34. Sharma, Priyanka, 'Intranasal Covid-19 Vaccines Will Be Game-Changers: Ella', *Mint*, 8 April 2022, https://bit.ly/3N6LR1b. Accessed on 25 October 2022.
35. 'First Nasal Vaccine against COVID-19 Supported by DBT-BIRAC Gets Emergency Use Authorization from India Drug Regulator DCGI', Press Information Bureau, Ministry of Science and Technology, 7 September 2022, https://bit.ly/3TGeynZ. Accessed on 25 October 2022.
36. Additionally, Bharat Immunologicals and Biologicals Limited, a central public sector unit in Bulandshahar, was granted ₹30 crore to enable the firm to produce 1.5 crore doses of the vaccine monthly. Haffkine Bio-Pharmaceutical Corporation Limited in Mumbai was given ₹65 crore to enable the Maharashtra government-owned firm to build 2 crore doses a month manufacture. The Haffkine Institute, originally set up in 1896 by Dr Waldemar Mordecai Haffkine, a Russian scientist and a student of Louis Pasteur, was the only body to make a vaccine for the 1897 plague, which killed several thousand Indians. Finally, Indian Immunologicals Limited in Hyderabad, originally set up by the National Dairy Development Board in 1982, was granted ₹60 crore.
37. 'PM Reviews Vaccine Development and Manufacturing Process at 3 Facilities', Press Information Bureau, Prime Minister's Office, 28 November 2020, https://bit.ly/3syyu0s. Accessed on 25 October 2022.
38. Nair, Lakshmipriya, 'How Glass Vial Makers are Girding to Boost Access to COVID-19 Vaccine', *Express Pharma*, 1 July 2020, https://bit.ly/3D8da6J. Accessed on 25 October 2022.

39. From an interview with Rajiv Nath, managing director, Hindustan Syringes and Medical Devices Limited, conducted by Aashish Chandorkar on 27 July 2022.
40. Ibid.
41. Singh, Karan Deep, 'The World Needs Syringes. He Jumped In to Make 5,900 per Minute', *The New York Times*, 5 March 2021, https://nyti.ms/3f6IoDj. Accessed on 25 October 2022.
42. Sharma, Sanchita, 'Learnings from Polio on How to Vaccinate 50 Million', *Hindustan Times*, 19 October 2020, https://bit.ly/3SztOlf. Accessed on 25 October 2022.
43. 'COVID-19 Vaccine Communication Strategy', Ministry of Health and Family Welfare, https://bit.ly/3FeTtwJ. Accessed on 25 October 2022.
44. 'English Rendering of PM's Address at the Laying of Foundation Stone of AIIMS Rajkot, Gujarat', Press Information Bureau, Prime Minister's Office, 31 December 2020, https://bit.ly/3zhVcNZ. Accessed on 25 October 2022.

Chapter 9: The Vaccines Roll Out

1. 'World's Largest Vaccination Programme Begins in India on January 16', *The Hindu*, 16 January 2022, https://bit.ly/3sATO5n. Accessed on 25 October 2022.
2. 'PM Launches Pan India Rollout of COVID-19 Vaccination Drive', Press Information Bureau, Prime Minister's Office, 16 January 2021, https://bit.ly/3zjiVNQ. Accessed on 25 October 2022.
3. Ibid.
4. @narendramodi, Twitter, 16 January 2021, 11.47 a.m., https://bit.ly/3NaLJ0H. Accessed on 25 October 2022.
5. 'Update on COVID-19 Vaccination', Press Information Bureau, Ministry of Health and Family Welfare, 16 January 2021, https://bit.ly/3VZRBOt. Accessed on 25 October 2022.
6. 'India Crosses a Landmark Milestone- More Than 1 Crore Vaccine Doses Administered Against COVID19', Press Information Bureau, Ministry of Health and Family Welfare, 19 February 2021, https://bit.ly/3DxmQsU. Accessed on 25 October 2022.
7. 'COVID 19 Vaccination Sessions Not Scheduled on Saturday and Sunday (27th & 28th Feb, 2021) in Wake of IT System Transition from Co-Win 1.0 to Co-Win 2.0', Press Information Bureau, Ministry of Health and Family Welfare', 26 February 2021, https://bit.ly/3syin2I. Accessed on 25 October 2022.
8. 'Registration for Next Phase of COVID19 Vaccination on Co-WIN2.0 Portal Will Open at 9:00 am on 1st March 2021 at www.Co-WIN.gov.in', Press

Information Bureau, Ministry of Health and Family Welfare, 28 February 2021, https://bit.ly/3zivNDH. Accessed on 25 October 2022.

9. Co-WIN, Ministry of Health and Family Welfare, https://bit.ly/3hcWl3j. Accessed on 4 November 2022.
10. Housel, Morgan, 'The Seduction of Pessimism', Collaborative Fund, 13 June 2017, https://bit.ly/3TDbKs0. Accessed on 25 October 2022.
11. @BDUTT, Twitter, 21 March 2020, 9.11 p.m., https://bit.ly/3gQOacw. Accessed on 28 October 2022.
12. 'India Will Take 12 Years to Vaccinate Entire Population, Reach Herd Immunity in 8 Years at Current Pace', *India Today*, 22 April 2021, https://bit.ly/3SJr0SK. Accessed on 25 October 2022.
13. Shrivastava, Rahul, 'Centre Approves Rs 3000 Cr Funds for Serum Institute, Rs 1500 Cr for Bharat Biotech to Ramp Up Vaccine Production', *India Today*, 20 April 2021, https://bit.ly/3FofFV1. Accessed on 28 October 2022.
14. 'Coronavirus (COVID-19) Vaccinations', Our World in Data, https://bit.ly/3U7iQoG. Accessed on 4 November 2022.
15. Barnagarwala, Tabassum, '9 Pvt Hospitals Corner 50% Doses, Raise Questions of Vaccine Equity and Access', *The Indian Express*, 5 June 2021, https://bit.ly/3FpetRA. Accessed on 28 October 2022.
16. 'Government of India Announces a Liberalised and Accelerated Phase 3 Strategy of Covid-19 Vaccination from 1st May', Press Information Bureau, Ministry of Health and Family Affairs, 19 April 2021, https://bit.ly/3U8eYDL. Accessed on 28 October 2022.
17. 'Serum's Adar Poonawalla Moves to London, Cites Threatening Phone Calls from Powerful People', *Business Today*, 2 May 2021, https://bit.ly/3sAizPd. Accessed on 28 October 2022.
18. 'Serum to Invest £240 m in UK Production', *Business Line*, 4 May 2021, https://bit.ly/3zpF7G1. Accessed on 28 October 2022.
19. Marpakwar, Chaitanya, 'Mumbai: BMC's Global Tender for Vaccine a Flop, All Nine Bids Junked', *The Times of India*, 5 June 2021, https://bit.ly/3sEcAZG. Accessed on 28 October 2022.
20. Nambiar, Nisha, 'No Response Yet to Maharashtra's Global Tender for Vaccines', *The Times of India*, 25 May 2021, https://bit.ly/3NdTYJi. Accessed on 28 October 2022.
21. 'English Rendering of PM's Address to the Nation', Press Information Bureau, Prime Minister's Office, 7 June 2021, https://bit.ly/3znabWK. Accessed on 28 October 2022.

Chapter 10: Vaccine Juggernaut: Lord Jagannatha's Irresistible Force Replayed

1. 'Serum Institute Produces over 100 Million Covishield Doses in June', *Business Standard*, 27 June 2021, https://bit.ly/3DOkwxX. Accessed on 28 October 2022.
2. 'Coronavirus (COVID-19) Vaccinations', Our World in Data, https://bit.ly/3zHTl5m. Accessed on 4 November 2022.
3. S., Suraj, 'The First Quarter Billion Doses: Looking Back and Ahead', *Swarajya*, 10 June 2021, https://bit.ly/3SJULmg. Accessed on 28 October 2022.
4. 'Coronavirus (COVID-19) Vaccinations', Our World in Data, https://bit.ly/3zHTl5m. Accessed on 4 November 2022.
5. S., Suraj, 'The Covid-19 "Vaccine Shortage": What Is Really Happening?', *Swarajya*, 13 April 2021, https://bit.ly/3DCf2pE. Accessed on 28 October 2022.
6. S., Suraj, 'Switching Tactics: Why India Must Temporarily Prioritise First Doses Mid-Wave', *Swarajya*, 28 April 2021, https://bit.ly/3feymA6. Accessed on 28 October 2022.
7. 'Co-WIN to Now Allow Bookings for 2nd Covishield Dose Only after 84 Days', *Hindustan Times*, 17 May 2021, https://bit.ly/3Dda15D. Accessed on 28 October 2022.
8. S., Suraj, 'How to Bulk Order Vaccines (And How Not To)', *Swarajya*, 14 May 2021, https://bit.ly/3W6Yc9I. Accessed on 28 October 2022.
9. 'Coronavirus (COVID-19) Vaccinations', Our World in Data, https://bit.ly/3ft7jkN. Accessed on 4 November 2022.
10. Ibid.
11. Co-WIN, Ministry of Health and Family Welfare, https://bit.ly/3zLe7AZ. Accessed on 4 November 2022.
12. Ibid.
13. 'Coronavirus (COVID-19) Vaccinations', Our World in Data, https://bit.ly/3ft7jkN. Accessed on 4 November 2022.

Chapter 11: Celebrating PM Modi's Birthday in Style

1. 'Countries in the World by Population', Worldometers, https://bit.ly/2v65eA9. Accessed on 28 October 2022.
2. Perappadan, Bindu Shajan, 'India Sets Record with 2.5 Crore COVID-19 Jabs in One Day', *The Hindu*, 18 September 2021, https://bit.ly/3NddnKi. Accessed on 28 October 2022.
3. @mansukhmandviya, Twitter, 17 September 2021, 9.40 a.m., https://bit.

ly/3gQoWuN. Accessed on 28 October 2022.

4. @mansukhmandviya, Twitter, 17 September 2022, 4.49 p.m., https://bit.ly/3ft0j7u. Accessed on 4 November 2022.
5. Perapaddan, Bindu Shajan, 'India Sets Record with 2.5 Crore COVID-19 Jabs in One Day', *The Hindu*, 18 September 2021, https://bit.ly/3NxizZU. Accessed on 4 November 2022.
6. @mansukhmandviya, Twitter, 18 September 2021, 4.01 p.m., https://bit.ly/3fzxru9. Accessed on 4 November 2022.
7. 'Update on COVID-19 Vaccine Availability in States/UTs', Press Information Bureau, Ministry of Health and Family Welfare, 16 September 2021, https://bit.ly/3TNww8q. Accessed on 28 October 2022.
8. Mullick, Jamie, 'Vaccination Boost Marks PM Modi's Birthday', *Hindustan Times*, 18 September 2021, https://bit.ly/3W7k3xL. Accessed on 28 October 2022.
9. Yasir, Sameer, 'India Boosts Its Covid Vaccine Drive with 25 Million Shots Given on Modi's Birthday', *The New York Times*, 17 September 2021, https://nyti.ms/3NdPT80. Accessed on 28 October 2022.
10. From an interview with Mansukh Mandaviya, cabinet minister, Health and Family Welfare, Government of India, conducted by Aashish Chandorkar on 28 April 2022 in Geneva.
11. 'Emotional Moment for Me, Says PM Modi on Record 2.5 Crore Vaccine Doses on His Birthday', *The Hindu*, 18 September 2021, https://bit.ly/3SLcSbw. Accessed on 28 October 2022.

Chapter 12: 2022: From Strength to Strength

1. 'India GDP Annual Growth Rate', Trading Economics, https://bit.ly/3U3KtiH. Accessed on 4 November 2022.
2. Callaway, Ewen, 'Heavily Mutated Omicron Variant Puts Scientists on Alert', *Nature*, 27 November 2021, https://go.nature.com/3Nd0no2. Accessed on 28 October 2022.
3. Dube, Mqondisi, 'To Reveal or Not to Reveal Omicron Origins, Botswana's Dilemma', Voice of America, 4 December 2021, https://bit.ly/3W7sbOT. Accessed on 28 October 2022.
4. 'Omicron COVID Variant Was in Europe before South African Scientists Detected and Flagged It to the World,' CBS News, 30 November 2021, https://cbsn.ws/3DBXvht. Accessed on 28 October 2022.
5. 'United States, Coronavirus (COVID-19)', Google News, https://bit.ly/3WIlFP1. Accessed on 4 November 2022.
6. Covid19Bharat, https://covid19bharat.org/, Accessed on 15 May 2022.

7. 'Omicron Was Less Severe in India Because of These 2 Reasons, Finds Study', *Mint*, 9 February 2022,https://bit.ly/3SHMLm4. Accessed on 28 October 2022.
8. Geddes, Linda, 'India versus Omicron: How the Country's Third COVID-19 Wave Might Unfold', Gavi, 17 January 2022, https://bit.ly/3W8Mco8. Accessed on 28 October 2022.
9. Mallapaty, Smriti, 'Fourth Dose of COVID Vaccine Offers Only Slight Boost against Omicron Infection', *Nature*, 23 February 2022, https://go.nature.com/3SKbiHd. Accessed on 28 October 2022.
10. Fleron, Addie, et al., 'The Gathering Storm: The Affordability Challenge of Endemic COVID-19', McKinsey & Company, 21 September 2022, https://mck.co/3fCnZq0. Accessed on 4 November 2022.
11. 'Dr. Mansukh Mandaviya reviews Public Health Preparedness to COVID19 and National COVID19 Vaccination Progress with States/UT', Press Information Bureau, Ministry of Health and Family Welfare, 2 January 2022, https://bit.ly/3feFNas. Accessed on 28 October 2022.
12. 'Over 40 Lakh Children Get Covid-19 Vaccine on First Day; Parents Say It's a Big Relief', *The Times of India*, 3 January 2022, https://bit.ly/3WmGbVd. Accessed on 28 October 2022.
13. @mygovindia, Twitter, 16 January 2022, 8.32 a.m., https://bit.ly/3sA9dmm. Accessed on 28 October 2022.
14. @narendramodi, Twitter, 16 January 2022, 11.41 a.m., https://bit.ly/3gOpqBM. Accessed on 28 October 2022.
15. @narendramodi, Twitter, 16 January 2022, 11.41 a.m., https://bit.ly/3DiOeJG. Accessed on 28 October 2022.
16. @narendramodi, Twitter, 16 January 2022, 11.41 a.m., https://bit.ly/3f7TE2p. Accessed on 28 October 2022.
17. @narendramodi, Twitter, 16 January 2022, 11.41 a.m., https://bit.ly/3U8caXb. Accessed on 28 October 2022.
18. Das, Sohini, 'Corbevax Becomes Third Covid vaccine to be Approved for Children in India', *Business Standard*, 22 February 2022, https://bit.ly/3Fl2UuA. Accessed on 28 October 2022.
19. From an interview with Dr Peter Hotez, dean for the National School of Tropical Medicine, Baylor College of Medicine Houston, United States, conducted by Abhinav Joshi, Aashish Chandorkar and Suraj Sudhir on 5 April 2022.
20. Ibid.
21. Ibid.
22. @mansukhmandviya, Twitter, 26 April 2022, 1. 35 p.m., https://bit.ly/3Dn3plo. Accessed on 28 October 2022.

23. Mashal, Mujib, and Karan Deep Singh, 'India's Rising Omicron Wave Brings a Grim Sense of Déjà Vu', *The New York Times*, 5 January 2022, https://nyti.ms/3FkVd7L. Accessed on 28 October 2022.
24. 'Is India Prepared for Omicron?', *The Economist*, 8 January 2022, https://econ.st/3sAnJKU. Accessed on 28 October 2022.
25. 'India May See 10 Lakh Covid Cases a Day by Jan-End: IISc-ISI Model', *The Economic Times*, 7 January 2022, https://bit.ly/3TpTj95. Accessed on 28 October 2022.
26. @agrawalmanindra, Twitter, 23 December 2021, 10.27 p.m., https://bit.ly/3W7o59n. Accessed on 28 October 2022.
27. @manujosephsan, Twitter, 23 May 2019, 9.40 a.m., https://bit.ly/3zmPSsS. Accessed on 28 October 2022.
28. @mansukhmandviya, Twitter, 14 March 2022, 1.48 p.m., https://bit.ly/3SFrt8t. Accessed on 28 October 2022.
29. Kaunain, Sheriff M., 'In a First, Centre Will Pay Rs 1,500 Crore to Reserve 30 Crore Doses of New Vaccine', *The Indian Express*, 4 June 2021, https://bit.ly/3zEoUN9. Accessed on 4 November 2022.
30. Co-WIN, Ministry of Health and Family Welfare, https://bit.ly/3NBLsnD. Accessed on 4 November 2022.
31. Ibid.
32. 'Vaccine Supply', COVID-19 Updates, Ministry of External Affairs, https://bit.ly/3DEPRBw. Accessed on 4 November 2022.

Chapter 13: An Achievement to Be Truly Proud Of

1. Bolt, Jutta, et al., '"Rebasing 'Maddison': New Income Comparisons and the Shape of Long-Run Economic Development', Maddison Project Database, 2018, https://bit.ly/3TDgz3q. Accessed on 15 November 2022.
2. 'Countries in the World by Population', Worldometers, https://bit.ly/2v65eA9. Accessed on 28 October 2022; 'Indian Age Structure', IndexMundi, https://bit.ly/2yKtES3. Accessed on 7 November 2022.
3. Co-WIN, Ministry of Health and Family Welfare, https://bit.ly/3hfbm4k. Accessed on 4 November 2022.
4. 'Coronavirus (COVID-19) Vaccinations', Our World in Data, https://bit.ly/3zIpo4Y. Accessed on 4 November 2022.
5. Co-WIN, Ministry of Health and Family Welfare, https://bit.ly/3hfbm4k. Accessed on 4 November 2022.
6. Ibid.
7. 'Coronavirus (COVID-19) Vaccinations', Our World in Data, https://bit.ly/3zIpo4Y. Accessed on 4 November 2022.

8. 'COVID-19 Vaccine Operational Guidelines', Ministry of Health and Family Welfare, Government of India, https://bit.ly/3Ufo5CB. Accessed on 31 October 2022.
9. Ibid.
10. 'COVID-19 Vaccine Operational Guidelines', Ministry of Health and Family Welfare, Government of India, https://bit.ly/3Ufo5CB. Accessed on 31 October 2022.
11. Reed, Tina, 'More than 1,700 U.S. Healthcare Workers Have Died from COVID-19, Nurses' Union Says', Fierce Healthcare, 28 September 2020, https://bit.ly/3SI7zKe. Accessed on 28 October 2022.
12. Chidambaram, Priya, 'Over 200,000 Residents and Staff in Long-Term Care Facilities Have Died from COVID-19', KFF, 3 February 2022, https://bit.ly/3TWD9Fa. Accessed on 28 October 2022.
13. Goldstein, Joshua R., and Ronald D. Lee, 'Demographic Perspectives on the Mortality of COVID-19 and Other Epidemics', *PNAS*, vol. 117, no. 36, 2020, pp. 22035–41.
14. From an interview with Mona, junior fellow, Observer Research Foundation, conducted by Aashish Chandorkar and Suraj Sudhir on 5 July 2022.
15. Monte, Lindsay M., 'Household Pulse Survey Shows Many Don't Trust COVID Vaccine, Worry About Side Effects', United States Census Bureau, 28 December 2021, https://bit.ly/3DnCjdH. Accessed on 31 October 2022.
16. From an interview with Pratyasha Rath, social science researcher, conducted by Aashish Chandorkar, Abhinav Joshi and Suraj Sudhir on 9 April 2022.
17. Co-WIN, Ministry of Health and Family Welfare, https://bit.ly/3hfbm4k. Accessed on 4 November 2022.
18. 'Total Population by Country 2022', World Population Review, https://bit.ly/3DCZX6c. Accessed on 4 November 2022.
19. Compiled from Government of India data sources as on 15 August 2022.

Chapter 14: Power of Public Digital Infrastructure

1. O'Reilly, 'Government as a Platform', *Innovations: Technology, Governance, Globalization*, vol. 6, no. 1, 2011, pp. 13–40.
2. 'PM's Address to the Nation on 15th August', Narendra Modi, 15 August 2014, https://bit.ly/3DL7hh7. Accessed on 31 October 2022.
3. From an interview with Ram Sewak Sharma, chief executive officer, National Health Authority, conducted by Aashish Chandorkar on 3 May 2022.
4. 'IT Minister Ravi Shankar Prasad Announces Launch of Grand Challenge for Strengthening the COVID Vaccine Intelligence Network (Co-WIN) System', Press Information Bureau, Ministry of Electronics and IT, 23

December 2020, https://bit.ly/3flOAYc. Accessed on 31 October 2022.

5. From discussions with the Ministry of Health and Family Welfare officials conducted by Aashish Chandorkar on 28 April 2022.
6. Ibid.
7. From an interview with Ram Sewak Sharma, chief executive officer, National Health Authority, conducted by Aashish Chandorkar on 3 May 2022.
8. Ibid.
9. From discussions with the Ministry of Health and Family Welfare officials, conducted by Aashish Chandorkar on 28 April 2022.
10. Ibid.
11. Ibid.
12. Thomas, Daniel, 'Can the US Crack Down on Fake Vaccination Cards?', BBC, 25 August 2021, https://bbc.in/3sKDnDC. Accessed on 31 October 2022.
13. Lenthang, Marlene, 'Two New York Nurses Made $1.5M in Fake Vaccine Card Scheme, Prosecutors Say', NBC News, 31 January 2022, https://nbcnews.to/3zpMltJ. Accessed on 31 October 2022.
14. 'Beware of Fraudulent Coronavirus Tests, Vaccines and Treatments', U.S. Food and Drug Administration', U.S. Food & Drug Administration, 3 February 2022, https://bit.ly/3DMidy5. Accessed on 31 October 2022.
15. Thrush, Glenn, 'The Justice Department Charged 21 People over Coronavirus-Related Fraud Schemes', *The New York Times*, 20 April 2022, https://nyti.ms/3NsqQ1e. Accessed on 31 October 2022.
16. Ibid.
17. From an interview with Ram Prasad, chief executive officer and co-founder, Final Mile Consulting, conducted by Aashish Chandorkar, Abhinav Joshi and Suraj Sudhir on 9 April 2022.
18. 'Thousands of Fake Covid-19 Certificates Uncovered in Switzerland', SWI, 23 December 2021, https://bit.ly/3gY1NGU. Accessed on 31 October 2022.
19. Méheut, Constant, and Elisabetta Povoledo, 'France Finds over 180,000 Fake Covid Passes, and Italy Makes Arrests in Suspected False Inoculations', *The New York Times*, 21 December 2021, https://nyti.ms/3FvTrk1. Accessed on 31 October 2022.
20. Ibid.
21. Pleschberger, Johannes, 'Austrian Police Investigate Fraud at Vienna COVID Vaccination Center', Euronews, 31 December 2021, https://bit.ly/3UctCJU. Accesed on 31 October 2022.
22. Bhalla, Kriti, '#StartupsVsCovid19: 7 Covid Vaccine Finder Apps Helping Indians Track and Book Jab Slots', Inc42, 7 May 2021, https://bit.ly/3WexOuB. Accessed on 31 October 2022.

23. Rana, Manjesh, 'Explained: How Digital Divide Impacts Young India's Covid-19 Vaccination Chances', *The Indian Express*, 7 June 2021, https://bit.ly/3zuSZ1X. Accessed on 31 October 2022.
24. 'Changes in Co-WIN App, Govt Restricts Vaccine Slot Info to Fight Bots and Alert Services, *India Today*, 7 May 2021, https://bit.ly/3DMlgDz. Accessed on 31 October 2022.
25. 'Allow States to Have Own Apps for Covid Vaccination, Says Maha CM', *Business Standard*, 8 May 2021, https://bit.ly/3FtYBNs. Accessed on 31 October 2022.
26. 'Allow States to Get Own App for Vaccination, Kejriwal Urges Centre, *The New Indian Express*, 10 May 2021, https://bit.ly/3NkQiFD. Accessed on 31 October 2022.
27. Agarwal, Surabhi, and Akshatha M., 'State Covid Apps Will Get to "Log into" Co-WIN', *The Economic Times*, 22 May 2021, https://bit.ly/3FvUfFz. Accessed on 31 October 2022.
28. Mukherji, Biman, 'India's Reliance on a Vaccine App Is Hindering Its Push for Herd Immunity', *Fortune*, 14 July 2021, https://bit.ly/3U9e3Th. Accessed 31 October 2022.
29. From an interview with Mona, junior fellow, Observer Research Foundation, conducted by Aashish Chandorkar and Suraj Sudhir on 5 July 2022.
30. From discussions with the Ministry of Health and Family Welfare officials, conducted by Aashish Chandorkar on 28 April 2022.
31. Ibid.
32. 'After Jharkhand, Chhattisgarh Replaces Modi's Photo on Vaccine Certificates With its Own CM', News18, 22 May 2021, https://bit.ly/3Nih01P. Accessed on 31 October 2022.
33. Philip, Shaju, 'Citizens' Duty to Respect PM, Says Kerala HC, Dismisses Plea against Modi Photo on Vaccination Certificate', *The Indian Express*, 21 December 2021, https://bit.ly/3zsJCzu. Accessed on 31 October 2022.
34. Ibid.
35. 'Prime Minister Shri Narendra Modi Inaugurates the Co-WIN Global Conclave', Press Information Bureau, Ministry of Health and Family Welfare, 5 July 2021, https://bit.ly/3gSA1M6. Accessed on 31 October 2022.
36. 'Dr. Harsh Vardhan addresses Co-WIN Global Conclave', Press Information Bureau, Ministry of Health and Family Welfare, 5 July 2021, https://bit.ly/3sI7ETk. Accessed on 31 October 2022.
37. From an interview with Ram Sewak Sharma, chief executive officer, National Health Authority, conducted by Aashish Chandorkar on 3 May 2022.
38. Pant, Manish, 'India's Fight against Pandemic Aided by Successful Co-WIN App', UNDP Asia and Pacific, 21 January 2022, https://bit.ly/3FvdoYh.

Accessed on 31 October 2022.

39. @AditiAnarayanan, Twitter, 20 July 2022, 5.48 p.m., https://bit.ly/3gZa11t. Accessed on 31 October 2022.
40. From an interview with Ram Sewak Sharma, chief executive officer, National Health Authority, conducted by Aashish Chandorkar on 3 May 2022.
41. 'The Digital India transformation', myGov blog, 3 June 2022, https://bit.ly/3sJw6Ut. Accessed on 31 October 2022.

Chapter 15: Vasudhaiva Kutumbakam

1. Moses, Jeffrey, *Oneness*, Random House Publishing, 2002, p. 12.
2. 'Inscriptions in Parliament House', Lok Sabha Secretariat, New Delhi, https://bit.ly/3TQk6wr. Accessed on 31 October 2022.
3. 'Text of PM's Address at the 75th United Nations General Assembly (UNGA) Session 2020', Press Information Bureau, Prime Minister's Office, 26 September 2020, https://bit.ly/3SKLPxj. Accessed on 31 October 2022.
4. Twohey, Megan, Keith Collins and Katie Thomas, 'With First Dibs on Vaccines, Rich Countries Have "Cleared the Shelves"', *The New York Times*, 15 December 2020, https://nyti.ms/3DMAWa0. Accessed on 31 October 2022.
5. 'Proceeds to GAVI from Donor Contributions & Pledges (2021–2025) as of 30 June 2022', Gavi, https://bit.ly/3fn4O3g. Accessed on 31 October 2022.
6. 'Phone Call between Prime Minister Shri Narendra Modi and H.E. Dr. Tedros Adhanom Ghebreyesus, Director General of the World Health Organisation (WHO)', Press Information Bureau, Prime Minister's Office, 11 November 2022, https://bit.ly/3sLvcXK. Accessed on 31 October 2022.
7. 'Prime Minister Chairs Meeting on the COVID-19 Pandemic Situation and Vaccine Delivery, Distribution and Administration', Press Information Bureau, Prime Minister's Office, 17 October 2020, https://bit.ly/3SQXaM4. Accessed on 31 October 2022.
8. 'Joint Statement on India-Bangladesh Virtual Summit', Press Information Bureau, Prime Minister's Office, 17 December 2020, https://bit.ly/3U8Fkp1. Accessed on 31 October 2022.
9. 'PM Modi Calls for Speedy Access to Covid Vaccines for Citizens Once Ready', *Business Standard*, 17 October 2020, https://bit.ly/3zqBcJ2. Accessed on 31 October 2022.
10. Poudel, Arjun, 'Nepal Asks India to Help Procure 20 Percent of Vaccines', *The Kathmandu Post*, 10 December 2020, https://bit.ly/3gVRt2q. Accessed on 31 October 2022.
11. Sharma, Kiran, 'Vaccine Powerhouse India Markets Affordable COVID Shots for Asia', Nikkei Asia, 24 December 2020, https://s.nikkei.com/3Ua6tYD.

Accessed on 31 October 2022.

12. Mohan, Geeta, 'India's Vaccine Diplomacy: 64 Foreign Envoys Visit Covid-19 Vaccine Facilities in Hyderabad', *India Today*, 9 December 2020, https://bit.ly/3Ucfgte. Accessed on 31 October 2022.
13. 'Vaccine Supply', Ministry of External Affairs, https://bit.ly/3h12EHa. Accessed on 31 October 2022.
14. 'Covid-19: India Dispatches 1.5 Lakh Doses of Covishield Vaccine as Gift to Bhutan', *The Times of India*, 20 January 2021, https://bit.ly/3gRcgUF. Accessed on 31 October 2022.
15. 'Press Release: Gift of 2nd consignment of the 'Made...', Embassy of India, Thimphu, Bhutan, 22 March 2021, https://bit.ly/3U8jUsb. Accessed on 31 October 2022.
16. 'Vaccine Supply', Ministry of External Affairs, https://bit.ly/3DAfKCE. Accessed on 4 November 2022.
17. Ibid.
18. Ibid.
19. 'Visit of Chief of Army Staff and Foreign Secretary to Myanmar (October 4-5, 2020)', Ministry of External Affairs, 5 October 2020, https://bit.ly/3Nnt15S. Accessed on 31 October 2022.
20. 'Vaccine Supply', Ministry of External Affairs, https://bit.ly/3TSUsXN. Accessed on 31 October 2022.
21. Ibid.
22. Ibid.
23. @jairbolsonaro, Twitter, 22 January 2021, 8.24 p.m., https://bit.ly/3DMEKrO. Accessed on 31 October 2022.
24. @miaamormottley, Twitter, 10 February 2021, 9.28 a.m., https://bit.ly/3zsOULm. Accessed on 31 October 2022.
25. Rawlins-Bentham, Julia, 'Minister Abrahams: Prison Security Not Compromised', Barbados Government Information Service, 2 January 2021, https://bit.ly/3Fqvpai. Accessed on 31 October 2022.
26. 'Barbados PM Requests PM Modi for Access to Oxford-AstraZeneca Vaccine Being Manufactured in India', *The Economic Times*, 23 January 2021, https://bit.ly/3DlKmHR. Accessed on 31 October 2022.
27. @rihanna, Twitter, 2 February 2021, 8.59 p.m., https://bit.ly/3FGx6k0. Accessed on 4 November 2022.
28. @miaamormottley, Twitter, 10 February 2021, 9.28 a.m., https://bit.ly/3DqrBTA. Accessed on 31 October 2022.
29. @miaamormottley, Twitter, 3 March 2021, 7.48 a.m., https://bit.ly/3fiatHK. Accessed on 31 October 2022.

30. @SkerritR, Twitter, 10 February 2021, 3.34 p.m. https://bit.ly/3gYLERO. Accessed on 31 October 2022.
31. @SkerritR, Twitter, 10 February 2021, 10.39 p.m., https://bit.ly/3Dq8Bok. Accessed on 31 October 2022.
32. @sidhant, Twitter, 10 February 2021, 4.31 p.m., https://bit.ly/3zuZBgN. Accessed on 31 October 2022.
33. 'Vaccine Supply', Ministry of External Affairs, https://bit.ly/3TSUsXN. Accessed on 31 October 2022.
34. 'General Council, 1-2 and 4 March 2021, Minutes of Meeting', World Trade Organization, 23 April 2021, https://bit.ly/3Wjg0hM. Accessed on 31 October 2022.
35. Pilla, Viswanath, 'Serum Institute Gets USFDA Nod to Export Novavax Covid Jab to US', *The Economic Times*, 15 July 2022, https://bit.ly/3SLN3rT. Accessed on 31 October 2022.
36. 'Vaccine Supply', Ministry of External Affairs, https://bit.ly/3TSUsXN. Accessed on 31 October 2022.
37. 'Vaccine Supply', Ministry of External Affairs, https://bit.ly/3TSUsXN. Accessed on 31 October 2022.
38. Fischer, William Weston, 'Patent: Law', Britannica, https://bit.ly/3zuuSQO. Accessed on 31 October 2022.
39. Naja, Abou, 'United Arab Emirates: History And Evolution of Intellectual Property', Mondaq, 18 August 2020, https://bit.ly/3DMsfwf. Accessed on 31 October 2022.
40. 'Inside WIPO', World Intellectual Property Organization, https://bit.ly/3U5PVRq. Accessed on 31 October 2022.
41. 'Intellectual Property: Protection and Enforcement', World Trade Organization, https://bit.ly/3gWbIgl. Accessed on 31 October 2022.
42. 'Part II — Standards Concerning the Availability, Scope and Use of Intellectual Property Rights', World Trade Organization, https://bit.ly/3gYP2w1. Accessed on 31 October 2022.
43. 'Declaration on the TRIPS Agreement and Public Health, Ministerial Conference, Fourth Session, Doha, 9–14 November 2001', World Trade Organization, 20 November 2001, https://bit.ly/3DLw0ly. Accessed on 31 October 2022.
44. 'Marrakesh Agreement Establishing the World Trade Organization', World Trade Organization, https://bit.ly/3DMd7Pp. Accessed on 31 October 2022.
45. 'Council for Trade-Related Aspects of Intellectual Property Rights, Minutes of Meeting', World Trade Organization, 3 February 2017, https://bit.ly/3Ufyiip. Accessed on 31 October 2022.
46. Tayor, Adam, 'In Secret Vaccine Contracts with Governments, Pfizer Took

Hard Line in Push for Profit, Report Says', *The Washington Post*, 19 October 2021, https://wapo.st/3NmFc34. Accessed on 31 October 2022.

47. Syam, Nirmalya, 'EU Proposals Regarding Article 31bis of the TRIPS Agreement in the Context of the COVID-19 Pandemic', Policy Brief, no. 100, August 2021, South Centre, https://bit.ly/3zuGMtP. Accessed on 31 October 2022.
48. Suneja, Kirtika, 'India appoints Brajendra Navnit as Ambassador to WTO', *The Economic Times*, 4 June 2020, https://bit.ly/3ff9VTf. Accessed on 31 October 2022.
49. From an interview with officials at the Permanent Mission of India to the World Trade Organization, Geneva, conducted by Aashish Chandorkar over March and April 2022.
50. Ibid.
51. 'Council for Trade-Related Aspects of Intellectual Property Rights, Waiver from Certain Provisions of the TRIPS Agreement for the Prevention, Containment and Treatment of Covid-19', World Trade Organization, 2 October 2020, https://bit.ly/3W9DNRk. Accessed on 31 October 2022.
52. 'Council for Trade-Related Aspects of Intellectual Property Rights, Minutes of Meeting', World Trade Organization, 16 February 2021, https://bit.ly/3SRnSnK. Accessed on 31 October 2022.
53. Ibid.
54. Kollewe, Julia, 'Pfizer Accused of Pandemic Profiteering as Profits Double', *The Guardian*, 8 February 2022, https://bit.ly/3Ue3KxA. Accessed on 31 October 2022.
55. 'Moderna Reports $18.5bn Total Revenue in Full-Year 2021', Pharmaceutical Technology, 25 February 2022, https://bit.ly/3TREj50. Accessed on 31 October 2022.
56. 'Statement from Ambassador Katherine Tai on the Covid-19 Trips Waiver', Office of the United States Trade Representative, 5 May 2021, https://bit.ly/3Dg6Qde. Accessed on 31 October 2022.
57. Silverman, Ed, 'A Compromise Is Reached on an Intellectual Property Waiver for Covid-19 Vaccines, But Does It Go Far Enough?', STAT, 15 March 2022, https://bit.ly/3SLPue1. Accessed on 31 October 2022.
58. @wto, Twitter, 16 March, 4.36 p.m., https://bit.ly/3NkAu5I. Accessed on 31 October 2022.
59. 'Director-General Okonjo-Iweala Hails Breakthrough on TRIPS COVID-19 Solution', World Trade Organization, 16 March 2022, https://bit.ly/3NjbUCp. Accessed on 31 October 2022.
60. 'Ministerial Conference, Twelfth Session, Geneva, 12-15 June 2022, Ministerial Decision on the TRIPS Agreement', World Trade Organization,

22 June 2022, https://bit.ly/3SRmW2P. Accessed on 31 October 2022.

Chapter 16: Taking It in Stride

1. 'PM Modi's address to the Nation on COVID-19 | 12th May 2020 | PMO', YouTube, 12 May 2020, https://bit.ly/3fp2oB1. Accessed on 31 October 2022.
2. Sagonowsky, Eric, 'Pfizer Eyes Higher Prices for COVID-19 Vaccine after the Pandemic Wanes: Exec, Analyst', Fierce Pharma, 23 February 2021, https://bit.ly/3ff3uj2. Accessed on 31 October 2022.
3. 'Training on handling, Storing and Transporting Pfizer BioNTech COVID-19 Vaccine COMIRNATY® (Tozinameran)', World Health Organization, 4 August 2021, https://bit.ly/3DlOTtR. Accessed on 31 October 2022.
4. Bickerton, Chris, 'Europe Failed Miserably With Vaccines. Of Course It Did', *The New York Times*, 17 May 2021, https://nyti.ms/3gMg5KI. Accessed on 31 October 2022.
5. Taylor, Adam, 'In Secret Vaccine Contracts with Governments, Pfizer Took Hard Line in Push for Profit, Report Says', *The Washington Post*, 19 October 2021, https://wapo.st/3NpfLxJ. Accessed on 31 October 2022.
6. Ibid.
7. Rizvi, Zain, 'Pfizer's Power', Public Citizen, 19 October 2021, https://bit.ly/3SOYDmb. Accessed on 31 October 2022.
8. Ibid.
9. Ibid.
10. From an interview with Ministry of Health and Family Welfare officials conducted by Aashish Chandorkar on 28 April 2022.
11. Ibid.
12. Gandhi-Mody, Priyam, *A Nation To Protect: Leading India through the Covid Crisis*, Rupa Publications, 2022, p. 144.
13. 'Training on Handling, Storing and Transporting Pfizer BioNTech COVID-19 Vaccine COMIRNATY® (Tozinameran)', World Health Organization, 4 August 2021, https://bit.ly/3DLPsP3. Accessed on 31 October 2022.
14. Kleinman, Zoe, 'How Will We Keep the Covid Vaccine at a Cold Enough Temperature?', BBC, 8 December 2020, https://bbc.in/3UdV2z0. Accessed on 31 October 2022.
15. Schaper, David, 'Transporting and Distributing Vaccines Will Be "Unprecedented" Logistical Challenge', NPR, 11 December 2020, https://n.pr/3fo6rOb. Accessed on 31 October 2022.
16. From an interview with Mansukh Mandaviya, minister of Health and Family

Welfare, Government of India, conducted by Aashish Chandorkar on 8 April 2022.
17. 'Vaccine Hesitancy: A Growing Challenge for Immunization Programmes', World Health Organization, 18 August 2015, https://bit.ly/3FzVmEi. Accessed on 31 October 2022.
18. From an interview with Ram Prasad, chief executive officer and co-founder, Final Mile Consulting, conducted by Aashish Chandorkar, Abhinav Joshi and Suraj Sudhir on 9 April 2022.
19. From an interview with Dr Raman Gangakhedkar, chief immunologist, Indian Council of Medical Research, conducted by Aashish Chandorkar on 2 April 2022.
20. From an interview with Pratyasha Rath, social science researcher, conducted by Aashish Chandorkar, Abhinav Joshi and Suraj Sudhir on 9 April 2022.
21. Ibid.
22. Ibid.
23. From an interview with Ram Prasad, chief executive officer and co-founder, Final Mile Consulting, conducted by Aashish Chandorkar, Abhinav Joshi and Suraj Sudhir on 9 April 2022.
24. 'Democracy Is in DNA of Every Indian: PM Modi', Narendra Modi, 26 June 2022, https://bit.ly/3Wkk2Xx. Accessed on 31 October 2022.
25. 'WHO Honours India's One Million All-Women ASHA Volunteers for "Outstanding" Work in Advancing Global Health', *The Print*, 22 May 2022, https://bit.ly/3NnASjS. Accessed on 31 October 2022.
26. 'Health Worker Rides Camel to Administer Covid-19 Vaccine Dose', *India Today*, 24 December 2021, https://bit.ly/3WkkhSr. Accessed on 31 October 2022.
27. From interviews with Ministry of Health and Family Welfare officials conducted by Aashish Chandorkar on 28 April 2022.
28. Bhat, Muzamil, 'Photos: Vaccination Drive Amidst Snow-Covered Mountains in Kashmir', *The Siasat Daily*, 29 January 2022, https://bit.ly/3FxY0dW. Accessed on 31 October 2022.
29. Azad, Shivani, 'Through Snow & Ice, 10 Hrs on Road: Race to Vax People Before Polls in Uttarakhand', *The Times of India*, 25 January 2022, https://bit.ly/3h0ciK9. Accessed on 31 October 2022.
30. 'In a First, Drone Delivers Covid Vaccines in Manipur', *The Times of India*, 5 October 2021, https://bit.ly/3DqfNAQ. Accessed on 31 October 2022.
31. From an interview with Dr Balram Bhargava, director general, Indian Council of Medical Research, conducted by Aashish Chandorkar on 24 April 2022.
32. Thakur, Aksheev, 'CSIR-NAL's "Octacopter" Drone Delivers Covid Vaccines

to Karnataka Village', *The Indian Express*, 10 November 2021, https://bit.ly/3NjgO2m. Accessed on 31 October 2022.

33. From interviews with Ministry of Health and Family Welfare officials conducted by Aashish Chandorkar on 28 April 2022.
34. Ibid.
35. Mittal, Ravi, and Oommen C. Kurian, 'Bringing the Covid-19 Vaccine to Every Hamlet: The Story of Raigarh', Observer Research Foundation, 2022, Special Report, no. 192, https://bit.ly/3WjEHe4. Accessed on 31 October 2022.
36. From an interview with Mona, junior fellow, Observer Research Foundation, conducted by Aashish Chandorkar and Suraj Sudhir on 5 July 2022.
37. From an interview with Kunal Agarwal, co-founder at Kool-ex, conducted by Aashish Chandorkar on 19 March 2022.
38. Wadhwa, Nilesh, 'Kool-ex Transports over 1 Crore Covid-19 Vaccine Doses in 30 Hours', Autocar Professional, 13 January 2021, https://bit.ly/3fnNQBN. Accessed on 31 October 2022.
39. From an interview with Kunal Agarwal, co-founder at Kool-ex, conducted by Aashish Chandorkar on 19 March 2022.
40. Sengupta, Joy, 'From January, Over 69 Crore Covishield Doses Transported from Pune Airport', *The Times of India*, 26 December 2021, https://bit.ly/3TSojzw. Accessed on 31 October 2022.
41. 'Remarks by President Biden on the Administration's COVID-19 Vaccination Efforts', The White House, 2 March 2021, https://bit.ly/3fo9VQL. Accessed on 31 October 2022.
42. 'The Defense Production Act of 1950: History, Authorities, and Considerations for Congress', Congressional Research Services, 20 November 2018, https://bit.ly/3sPmSG8. Accessed on 31 October 2022.
43. 'How the US Locked Up Vaccine Materials Other Nations Urgently Need', *The Economic Times*, 7 May 2021, https://bit.ly/3TTu2Fi. Accessed on 31 October 2022.
44. Ghoshal, Aniruddha, 'Indian Vaccine Maker Asks US to Ease Export Curbs', 16 April 2021, AP News, https://bit.ly/3fm6dqQ. Accessed on 31 October 2022.
45. 'Bharat Biotech Inks Deal with ViroVax for Adjuvant to Covaxin', *The Indian Express*, 6 October 2020, https://bit.ly/3gVMTRA. Accessed on 31 October 2022.
46. Bhargava, Balram, *Going Viral*, Rupa Publications, 2021, p. 116.
47. From interviews with officials in the Prime Minister's Office conducted by Aashish Chandorkar on 22 March 2022.
48. 'US Removes Defense Production Act Ratings on AstraZeneca, Novavax,

Sanofi Vaccines', *The Print*, 4 June 2021, https://bit.ly/3Dp9gqg. Accessed on 31 October 2022.

49. Thacker, Teena, 'Relief for Serum Institute of India as US Lifts Curbs on Vaccine Inputs', *The Economic Times*, 5 June 2021, https://bit.ly/3gWCepU. Accessed on 31 October 2022.
50. Bown, Chad P., 'The US Was Quick to Produce COVID-19 Vaccines. Then It Fell Behind', Peterson Institute of International Economics, 21 June 2022, https://bit.ly/3sKOyMs . Accessed on 31 October 2022.
51. 'WHO Issues Emergency Use Listing for Eighth COVID-19 Vaccine', World Health Organization, 3 November 2021, https://bit.ly/3sLpG7g. Accessed on 31 October 2022.
52. Sinha, Saurabh, 'UK Accepts Covishield, But Indians to Quarantine', *The Times of India*, 23 September 2021, https://bit.ly/3DqCXXI. Accessed on 31 October 2022.
53. From Aashish Chandorkar's meeting with PM Narendra Modi, 7 Lok Kalyan Marg, 16 July 2021.

Chapter 17: Leadership: Doing the Right Things

1. From interviews with unnamed officials from the Prime Minister's Office conducted by Aashish Chandorkar on 20 March 2022.
2. From an interview with Balram Bhargava, director general, Indian Council for Medical Research, conducted by Aashish Chandorkar on 22 April 2022.
3. From an interview with Shekhar Mande, retired director general, Council of Scientific and Industrial Research, conducted by Aashish Chandorkar on 10 May 2022.
4. From an interview with Dr V.K. Paul, chairperson, NITI Aayog, conducted by Aashish Chandorkar on 2 May 2022.
5. 'English Rendering of PM's Speech at Launch of PM Ayushman Bharat Health Infrastructure Mission in Varanasi', Press Information Bureau, Prime Minister's Office, 25 October 2021, https://bit.ly/3ffaI6E. Accessed on 31 October 2022.
6. 'Budget 2021 -2022, Speech of Nirmala Sitharaman, Minister of Finance', 1 February 2021', India Budget, https://bit.ly/3fh9Gaf. Accessed on 31 October 2022.
7. From interview with officials of Ministry of Health and Family Welfare conducted by Aashish Chandorkar on 22 April 2022.
8. 'English Rendering of PM's Speech at Launch of PM Ayushman Bharat Health Infrastructure Mission in Varanasi', Press Information Bureau, Prime Minister's Office, 25 October 2021, https://bit.ly/3ffaI6E. Accessed on 31 October 2022.

9. 'One Health Consortium', Press Information Bureau, Ministry of Science and Technology, 9 December 2021, https://bit.ly/3SRJYH5. Accessed on 31 October 2022.
10. Ibid.
11. From an interview with Shekhar Mande, retired director general, Council of Scientific and Industrial Research, conducted by Aashish Chandorkar on 10 May 2022.
12. From an interview with Ram Sewak Sharma, chief executive officer, National Health Authority, conducted by Aashish Chandorkar on 3 May 2022.
13. Ibid.
14. 'Govt Plans to Repurpose Co-WIN for Its Universal Immunisation Programme', *The Hindu*, 27 May 2022, https://bit.ly/3U9vcfz. Accessed on 31 October 2022.
15. From an interview with Ram Sewak Sharma, chief executive officer, National Health Authority, conducted by Aashish Chandorkar on 3 May 2022.
16. From an interview with Shekhar Mande, retired director general, Council of Scientific and Industrial Research, conducted by Aashish Chandorkar on 10 May 2022.
17. Mande, Shekhar, 'Is SARS-CoV-2 Airborne?', Council of Scientific and Industrial Research, https://bit.ly/3gWaUIr. Accessed on 31 October 2022.
18. Mascarenhas, Anuradha, 'CSIR Study to Explore Possibility of Airborne Transmission of Coronavirus', *The Indian Express*, 7 August 2020, https://bit.ly/3NiWKgw. Accessed on 31 October 2022.
19. Lewis, Dyani, 'Why the WHO Took Two Years to Say COVID Is Airborne', *Nature*, 6 April 2022, https://go.nature.com/3DLGLnW. Accessed on 31 October 2022.
20. 'Covid-19: Government Guidelines on ACs, Coolers and Fans', *The Times of India*, 25 April 2020, https://bit.ly/3fonVKo. Accessed on 31 October 2022.
21. 'CSIR Guidelines on Ventilation of Residential and Office Buildings for SARS-CoV-2 Virus Version 2.0 (2022)', Council of Scientific and Industrial Research, https://bit.ly/3zvbjbf. Accessed on 31 October 2022.
22. From an interview with Shekhar Mande, retired director general, Council of Scientific and Industrial Research, conducted by Aashish Chandorkar on 10 May 2022.
23. 'Fact Sheet: Quad Leaders' Summit', The White House, 24 September 2021, https://bit.ly/3TTxKPe. Accessed on 31 October 2022.
24. 'Vaccine Handover to Thailand under the Quad Vaccine Partnership', U.S. Embassy & Consulate in Thailand, 21 April 2022, https://bit.ly/3fpb8aj. Accessed on 31 October 2022.

25. 'Fact Sheet: Quad Leaders' Summit', The White House, 24 September 2021, https://bit.ly/3TTxKPe. Accessed on 31 October 2022.
26. 'Remarks of Senator John F. Kennedy, Convocation of the United Negro College Fund, Indianapolis, Indiana, April 12, 1959', John F. Kennedy Presidential Library and Museum, https://bit.ly/3Wb9tG9. Accessed on 31 October 2022.

Chapter 18: Aatmanirbhar Bharat

1. Basu, Nayanima, '"Look beyond Ukraine, World Threw Afghanistan under the Bus": Jaishankar Reminds Europe', *The Print*, 26 April 2022, https://bit.ly/3TPyvJp. Accessed on 31 October 2022.
2. 'PM Delivers the Keynote Address at the National Launch Ceremony of "Azadi Ke Amrit Mahotsav se Swarnim Bharat Ke Ore"', Narendra Modi, 20 January 2022, https://bit.ly/3h1jtli. Accessed on 31 October 2022.
3. @ANI, Twitter, 24 November 2015, 6.33 p.m., https://bit.ly/3DqhYob. Accessed on 31 October 2022.

INDEX